PREGNANCY
WEEK BY WEEK

Understand the changes and chart the progress of
you and your baby with this essential handy guide

Dr Jane MacDougall

hamlyn

An Hachette UK company
www.hachette.co.uk

First published in Great Britain in 2011 by
Carroll & Brown Publishers Limited

This edition published in 2015 by Hamlyn,
a division of Octopus Publishing Group Ltd
Carmelite House
50 Victoria Embankment
London EC4Y 0DZ
www.octopusbooks.co.uk

ISBN 978-0-600-63144-6

A CIP catalogue record for this book is available from the
British Library.

Printed and bound in China

10 9 8 7 6 5 4 3 2 1

Art Director Chrissie Lloyd
Managing Art Editor Emily Cook
Editorial Assistance Alison Howard
Photography Jules Selmes

Illustrations
Amanda Williams

Suppliers
Thanks to Mothercare, for equipment shown p38, p54 (blankets)
and p56.

Photolibrary.com
Jacket, p6, p14, p20, p22, p42 bottom left, p62, p74, p76, p82, p87
and p88.

Science Photo Library
P8 Prof. P. Motta/Dept. of Anatomy/University "La Sapienza",
Rome/Science Photo Library and p22 Ian Hooton/Science
Photo Library.

CONTENTS

FOREWORD

Pregnancy Week by Week is the best companion any expectant mother can have. Although every pregnancy is unique, the book covers the experiences most women are likely to have over these nine vital months, as well as showing how an unborn baby develops in the uterus from week to week. There is also a 'dates for your diary' planner at the bottom of every week page on which to jot down your antenatal appointments, test dates and results, and record any important tasks and events. This can help ensure both you and your baby's good health and to prepare for your baby's arrival.

The book's convenient size means you can carry it around with you to your appointments – or when you are just out and about. Its spiral binding enables you to stand the book up on your dresser or desktop, so that you can see at a glance the changes to your baby taking place each week as well as your appointments diary, if you so desire.

Inside you will find accurate and accessible information, reflecting current medical opinion on a variety of subjects ranging from preconception care, how to cope with

common symptoms of pregnancy, nutritional and exercise advice, the latest medical and diagnostic tests, information on where and how to have your baby, what to pack for the hospital and how to decorate your baby's nursery.

The text contains many headings and information boxes, which make it easy for you to dip in to find the subject you require, without reading the whole book cover to cover. Your baby's weekly progress is imagined in specially commissioned illustrations augmented by information on his probable size.

Pregnancy Week by Week is the ideal self-purchase for anyone planning a family and a great gift for those already expecting, as well as for prospective grandparents. It aims to provide concise, reassuring advice leading to a healthy and happy pregnancy and a healthy newborn – with the added satisfaction of being able to view the new baby's development.

USEFUL CONTACT DETAILS

As a quick and easy reference, fill in the following information and try to keep it as up to date as possible.

This book belongs to
Name

Address

Telephone number

Hospital number

Blood group

Allergies:

Medications

Birth partner
Name

Telephone number

Hospital
Name

Address

Telephone number

Consultant
Name

Address

Telephone number

GP
Name

Address

Telephone number

Midwife
Name

Address

Telephone number

Childbirth class instructor
Name

Address

Telephone number

Car/taxi service
Name

Telephone number

Pharmacy
Name

Address

Telephone number

PLANNING TO CONCEIVE

Fundamental to trying for a baby is evaluating your lifestyle and that of your partner, and making adjustments to ensure that both of you are in the best possible shape. Ideally, this should be done at least one month, but preferably three months, beforehand.

Eliminate or decrease harmful substances

Smoking, alcohol and caffeine can be harmful to an expectant woman, her fetus and newborn (see page 13). Therefore, it is vital that both partners stop smoking and cut down on alcohol and caffeine intake when trying to conceive.

Adjust diet and weight

At least one month, and preferably three, prior to conception you should make certain you are eating a diet rich in essential nutrients (see page 9) and low in fatty or sugary foods. You should also supplement your diet with foods containing folic acid (see page 9). Being overweight can cause problems during pregnancy, while being underweight can affect your reproductive cycle

(see page 8) and chances of conception. Check with your doctor to see if your weight needs adjusting. Generally, it's not a good idea to diet during pregnancy, because your unborn baby may suffer from a lack of nutrients essential for his development.

Work on your emotional well-being

Pregnancy, birth and parenthood will deeply and irrevocably affect your relationships, especially that with your partner. Most parents are overwhelmed by the joys and challenges a new baby presents, though some may suffer from worry, resentment and even depression. Use the time before conception to talk with your partner and discuss any doubts or insecurities.

Adjust your contraception

If you are using the pill or an IUD, switch to the diaphragm, cap or condoms about three months before you plan to conceive. This will ensure you have at least one normal menstrual cycle before you become pregnant. If you conceive while you are still using the pill or an IUD, talk to your doctor.

Seek genetic counselling

If there is a history of hereditary diseases, such as haemophilia or cystic fibrosis in your family, or if you know that you and your partner have incompatible blood types (see page 22), consider seeing a genetic counsellor for advice before you conceive. Depending on ethnic background, other tests may be offered.

Get into shape
Your body will undergo many changes during pregnancy, so use the time before you conceive to attain a certain level of fitness (see page 29). Being fit will also help you have an easier delivery.

Mum-to-be

Ideally, you should be in the best possible shape for conception and future parenthood, having stopped smoking, overindulging in alcohol and avoided unnecessary medications. You also should have moved away from, or be planning to leave, any potentially hazardous work situation (see page 44). If you or anyone in your immediate family suffers from a pre-existing disease, discuss with your doctor any possible risks this may pose to a pregnancy.

BASAL BODY TEMPERATURE CHART

Dates covered: Day _____ Month _____ Year _____ to Day _____ Month _____ Year _____

Cycle Day	1	2	3	4	5	6	7	8	9	10	11	12	13	14	15	16	17	18	19	20	21	22	23	24	25	26	27	28
Weekday																												
Date																												
Time																												
37.3°C																												
37.2°C																												
37.1°C																												
37.0°C																												
36.9°C																												
36.8°C																												
36.7°C																												
36.6°C																												
36.5°C																												
36.4°C																												
36.3°C																												
36.2°C																												
36.1°C																												
36.0°C																												

Either photocopy three copies of this chart or print off a similar one from the internet. Mark a dot next to your temperature on each day of the three months and join the dots. You will soon see two patterns of temperature emerging – lower and higher. You are more likely to conceive when your temperature is higher and it is then that you should have more frequent intercourse.

Basal body temperature

Your basal body temperature can be measured on a basal body thermometer and charted to detect rises in temperature – the most likely time of ovulation. Now your temperature should hover near the 36.6°C mark but, hopefully, this will rise next week.

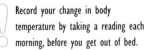
Record your change in body temperature by taking a reading each morning, before you get out of bed.

DATES FOR YOUR DIARY

MONDAY	TUESDAY	WEDNESDAY	THURSDAY	FRIDAY	SATURDAY/SUNDAY

FERTILISATION

During your reproductive life, your uterus prepares for pregnancy every month, in the form of your menstrual cycle. Day one of your cycle is the first day of menstrual bleeding, when the lining (endometrium) of your uterus is shed. When bleeding stops, the endometrium is rebuilt. At about day five an ovum, or egg, starts to mature inside a fluid-filled sac (the follicle) in one of the two ovaries situated close to your fallopian tubes. In a 28-day cycle, at about day 14 when the follicle is mature, it ruptures and releases the egg. The ruptured follicle becomes the corpus luteum. This structure makes the hormone progesterone, which plays a vital role in helping your body adapt to pregnancy and in the early development of the embryo, if fertilisation occurs. If you are to conceive, during ejaculation millions of your partner's sperm travel from your vagina to the fallopian tube. A few hundred sperm will make it to a waiting egg and release an enzyme that will allow one of them to penetrate its protective coating. This is the moment of fertilisation. Should one of your partner's sperm penetrate your egg, all other sperm are prevented from doing so.

CONCEIVING TWINS

There are two types of twins: identical and non-identical or fraternal. Identical twins develop from the fertilisation of a single egg by a single sperm. The egg divides into a zygote (two cells) then separates into two zygotes. These zygotes continue dividing in the normal way to eventually produce two fetuses with identical genes. Identical twins may or may not share a placenta and amniotic sac, but each twin has his own umbilical cord. Non-identical twins develop when two eggs are fertilised by two separate sperm. Each fetus has his own placenta and individual genetic make-up.

Identical twins

Non-identical twins

Sperm meet egg
The tiny sperm are dwarfed by the ovum; here they attempt to pierce the zona pellucida, the ovum's protective covering.

Mum-to-be

Ovulation usually occurs 14 days prior to your next period, so, if you have a 28-day cycle, day 14 is when you are most likely to conceive. On this, or any adjusted date (due to the length of your cycle), you should start having regular sex with your partner. The body of this 'lucky' sperm dissolves and its nucleus, containing your partner's genetic material, fuses with that of the egg, which contains yours.

Because ovulation usually occurs around day 14, a missed menstrual period two weeks later, should indicate pregnancy. Traditionally, pregnancy is dated from the first day of your last menstrual period (LMP). However, if you are said to be four weeks pregnant (that is, it is four weeks after your LMP), your fetus' age and the period of gestation is only two weeks.

Baby

The sex of your baby is determined by two of the 46 chromosomes that make up his or her genetic blueprint. The egg and sperm each carry one. The egg has an X chromosome but the sperm has either an X or a Y chromosome. If an X-bearing sperm fertilises the egg, you will have a girl; if the sperm carries a Y chromosome, you will have a boy. Therefore, the father determines his baby's gender.

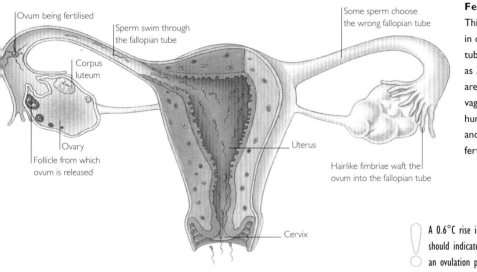

Ovum being fertilised

Sperm swim through the fallopian tube

Corpus luteum

Ovary

Follicle from which ovum is released

Some sperm choose the wrong fallopian tube

Uterus

Hairlike fimbriae waft the ovum into the fallopian tube

Cervix

Fertilisation

This usually takes place in one of the fallopian tubes. Although as many as 300 million sperm are ejaculated into the vagina, only a few hundred reach the tube, and only one will fertilise the egg.

A 0.6°C rise in temperature this week should indicate ovulation. Confirm with an ovulation predictor kit.

DATES FOR YOUR DIARY

MONDAY	TUESDAY	WEDNESDAY	THURSDAY	FRIDAY	SATURDAY/SUNDAY

HEALTHY EATING

Your baby receives all her nourishment via your bloodstream, so it's important that you maintain a healthy diet. Any extra calories – approximately 300 per day (should you be underweight) – would only be necessary in the last three months when your baby is putting on fat. The need for protein, which is vital for creating new tissue, more than doubles during pregnancy, as does the requirement for calcium, necessary for baby's bone and teeth formation – at least in the last three months.

Iron is essential for the formation of haemoglobin, the oxygen-carrying pigment in red blood cells, and your baby's increasing volume of blood relies on a healthy supply of iron from your diet. Lack of iron – as well as vitamin B_{12} and folic acid, which aid the development of healthy blood cells – may result in anaemia.

Folic acid is vital for preventing spina bifida, a neural tube disorder, and you should take a supplement containing 400 mcg folic acid starting three months prior to conception. Talk to your doctor about antenatal vitamins and continued consumption of folic acid to ensure you are getting all the important nutrients you need. Some prescribed medications reduce the absorption of folic acid, so make sure you check with your doctor, who may prescribe a higher dose.

Fluid intake

To keep your skin looking good and to maintain a healthy circulation and digestion, it's also important to drink at least eight (225 ml) glasses of fluids – preferably water – a day. During pregnancy, the volume of blood flowing around your body doubles so you need to maintain a high fluid intake.

SOURCES OF ESSENTIAL NUTRIENTS

Vitamin A	Dairy products, eggs, oily fish, yellow, orange and green vegetables
Vitamin B_1	Whole grains, brewer's yeast, nuts, legumes, green leafy vegetables, pork
Vitamin B_2	Whole grains, green vegetables, eggs
Vitamin B_3	Whole grains, brewer's yeast, oily fish, eggs, milk
Vitamin B_5	Eggs, legumes, nuts, whole grains, avocados
Vitamin B_6	Whole grains, brewer's yeast, potatoes, mushrooms, extra-lean meat
Vitamin B_{12}	Eggs, meat, oysters, milk
Folic acid	Leafy green vegetables, oranges, legumes
Vitamin C	Citrus fruits, strawberries, sweet peppers, tomatoes, potatoes
Vitamin D	Fortified milk, oily fish (tinned sardines), margarine, egg yolk, sunlight
Vitamin E	Vegetable oils, wheat germ, nuts, sunflower seeds, broccoli
Calcium	Dairy products, canned sardines and salmon including bones, leafy green vegetables, legumes
Iron	Red meat, legumes, eggs, leafy green vegetables
Zinc	Wheat germ, wheat bran, nuts, onions, oysters, extra-lean meat, poultry

Snacking

Avoid fatty, sugary foods such as biscuits; munch on fresh fruit and vegetables. Fruit is generally refreshing and contains fibre, which helps prevent constipation, a common complaint in pregnancy (see page 46).

Mum-to-be

Roughly seven days after fertilisation, the morula – a solid ball of cells – implants in the lining of your uterus (the endometrium). As the ball of cells matures it becomes a blastocyst, secreting substances that trigger profound changes in your body, including the halting of the menstrual cycle.

Baby

After an egg has been fertilised, conception has been achieved and cells begin to multiply at a tremendous rate. In just seven days, a single cell transforms into a ball of hundreds. Although you can't make out much organisation – even under a microscope – the cells are already grouping in a pre-determined way. Some are destined to become the embryo, others to form the support structures (villi and placenta) that will nurture it. How this happens is still largely a mystery, but we do know that it involves a complex series of interactions.

The blastocyst, a hollow, fluid-filled ball of cells, burrows into the top part of the uterus. This happens between days four and seven, although it may not be firmly implanted until day ten. Cells from the outer coating of the blastocyst project root-like attachments, called villi, into the endometrium. Villi allow an exchange of nutrients and waste between your bloodstream and the developing embryo. This connection will eventually mature into the placenta, the organ that will feed and protect your growing baby in the months ahead. Meanwhile, the lining of the uterus grows over the blastocyst, sealing it in.

From egg to embryo

The fertilised egg divides within hours to give a two-cell zygote, which continues to divide and subdivide until it forms a solid ball the size of a pinhead, the morula. After about four days, the morula transforms itself into a fluid-filled ball of approximately 100 cells, the blastocyst, from which the placenta and embryo will develop.

Making love every two days this week (and the last) will increase your chances of conceiving.

DATES FOR YOUR DIARY

MONDAY	TUESDAY	WEDNESDAY	THURSDAY	FRIDAY	SATURDAY/SUNDAY

MENU PLANNING

Eating well does not mean worrying about calorie consumption, rather it means being aware of the quality and nutritional content of the foods you eat. Some nutrients are essential for a healthy pregnancy (see page 10), and as long as you make sure you have the recommended daily intake of these, your body should be able to adjust to the demands of a pregnancy quite happily.

It is important to eat a wide variety of foods during pregnancy, as foods supply different nutrients in varying quantities. Citrus fruits, for example, provide vitamin C, which aids iron absorption and cell function, and sardines contain vitamin D, vital for sustaining the immune system.

Eating small meals frequently throughout the day will help you to digest food more effectively and give you more consistent energy. Eating small meals may also be helpful if you suffer from morning sickness.

Below is a suggested menu for one day (annotated to show what nutrients the foods provide). This is only a guide, so try to vary it with similar alternatives to suit your own tastes.

FOODS TO AVOID

- High fat, sugary foods. These lack nutrients and only provide what are known as 'empty calories'.
- Unpasteurised milk and soft and blue-veined cheeses, packaged salads, cooked food chilled for reheating and pâtés. These have all been found to contain listeria, a bacteria that in rare cases can cause miscarriage or stillbirth.
- Raw or undercooked meats and poultry. These may cause toxoplasmosis – a disease that can bring about fetal brain damage and blindness.
- Raw and undercooked eggs and poultry. They may contain potentially dangerous salmonella bacteria.
- Liver. Too much vitamin A can be harmful in pregnancy.
- More than two portions of oily fish a week.

DAILY MENU

Breakfast
Eggs and whole wheat bread (B and E vitamins, fibre, iron)
Yogurt flavoured with fruits (calcium, vitamin C, fibre)
A glass of orange juice (vitamin C and fluids)

Morning snack
Whole wheat bread (fibre) with peanut butter (protein, fibre, vitamin E, folic acid)
Bananas (potassium)
A glass of milk (protein, calcium)

Lunch
Broccoli and cheese soup (folic acid, calcium, protein)
Sardines (calcium, vitamin D)
Potatoes (vitamin C, fibre, carbohydrates)

Afternoon snack
Sticks of raw vegetables, such as carrots and celery (vitamins, minerals)
Whole wheat crackers (fibre, carbohydrates)

Evening snack
Cheese and crackers (calcium and fibre)
A glass of milk (protein, calcium)

Dinner
Chicken (protein)
Whole grain rice (carbohydrates, fibre)
Vegetables (vitamins, minerals)
Fresh fruit (fibre, vitamins, natural sugars)

Mum-to-be

If you suspect you may be pregnant, only a blood test will give you the most accurate result at this stage because home pregnancy tests are unable to detect the very small quantities of the pregnancy hormone, human chorionic gonadotropin (hCG), which the placenta has now secreted into your blood. As you wait to see whether or not your period arrives, you may experience a few pregnancy symptoms similar to premenstrual ones, such as queasiness or heavy breasts.

Baby

The blastocyst arrives in the uterus. Comprising hundreds of cells, it begins to attach itself to the uterine wall. The cells grow into the chorionic villi, which will later become the placenta. Released enzymes then pierce the uterine lining, causing tissue breakdown and providing nourishing blood cells on which the chorionic villi feed. The implantation process takes about 13 days.

Once the blastocyst implants, its cells begin to separate into layers. The top layer becomes the embryo and amniotic cavity and the lower layer becomes the yolk sac. The yolk sac will manufacture blood cells for the embryo until its own bone marrow is ready to take over the job (see page 65). The embryo further divides into three layers, as below.

Development of the embryo

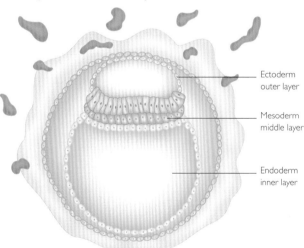

Ectoderm outer layer

Mesoderm middle layer

Endoderm inner layer

Cell sandwich

Here you see the embryonic cell layers. The inner layer develops into the lungs, liver, bladder, thyroid gland, gastrointestinal system and pancreas; the middle layer forms the skeleton, muscles, heart, circulation and kidneys; the outer layer will become the brain and nervous system, teeth and skin.

You may want to try an over-the-counter pregnancy test to see if you have conceived.

DATES FOR YOUR DIARY

MONDAY	TUESDAY	WEDNESDAY	THURSDAY	FRIDAY	SATURDAY/SUNDAY

POTENTIAL HAZARDS

Smoking

Smoking should be avoided. It can result in preterm delivery, miscarriage, placenta praevia, placental abruption and preterm rupture of the membranes. Once your baby is born, it may also lead to Sudden Infant Death Syndrome (SIDS). Secondary smoking, which is if your partner or any other household member smokes, will affect your baby's health leading to respiratory problems and even SIDS. Even passive smoking (being in a smoke-filled environment) is very dangerous, as it could result in low birth weight and developmental disorders. It's not recommended to take nicotine substitutions and anti-smoking medications while pregnant.

Food-borne infections

Certain foods (see page 12), as well as preparation techinques, can result in harmful organisms damaging your unborn baby as well as giving you food poisoning. Wash your hands and all equipment thoroughly before and after cooking, use separate cutting boards for meats and make sure food is refrigerated properly. Do not handle cat litter trays.

Household cleaning products

Cleaning products used in the home, and even some personal care products, can contain chemicals that are dangerous to a developing fetus. Avoid contact with pesticides and highly toxic products, such as oven cleaner, and always ventilate rooms well while cleaning.

Alcohol

It's best not to drink alcohol at all, although if you have the occasional drink – no more than one or two units a week – you will probably not harm your baby. Drinking excessively can lead to miscarriage, low birth weight, mental retardation, neurological disorders, behavioural problems, learning deficiencies, Fetal Alcohol Syndrome and physical deformities. A single unit of alcohol would be 85 ml of wine (a small glass is equal to 125 ml or 1½ units); two pints of ordinary-strength lager, ale or beer (some continental varieties are stronger); a 25 ml shot of spirits or a 50 ml aperitif. An alcopop usually contains 1½ units. Drink alcohol only when eating.

Caffeine

Too much caffeine reduces the absorption of nutrients and can result in low birth weight or miscarriage. In addition to tea and coffee, caffeine is found also in colas, energy drinks and chocolate, as well as in cold-and-flu remedies and some painkillers. Limit your intake to less than 200 mg a day (1–2 small coffees a day).

Medications and drugs

Few medicines have been established as safe to use while pregnant, so always discuss the pros and cons with your doctor if ever you are prescribed medication, including over-the-counter painkillers. If you are already on medication, say for a chronic condition or illness, such as diabetes or high blood pressure, make sure you dicuss the medication with your doctor in case a change in treatment is needed or the dosage needs to be adjusted. For short-term illnesses like colds, ask the pharmacist what treatment is best, since most over-the-counter medicine isn't advisable when pregnant.

Mum-to-be

An over-the-counter pregnancy test now may be able to confirm that you are pregnant, which you should suspect after missing a period. If test results are negative, you may want to repeat the test a few days later, particularly if your period has still not arrived. If the test is positive, think about whether you tell people now or wait until after the first trimester (after week 12), when complications are less likely.

Your breasts may be feeling fuller and more tender and you may suffer from fatigue. If you start to feel a little nauseous – particularly in the morning – try eating smaller meals and milder-tasting foods to see if that will settle your stomach. Of course you may not be feeling any different. However, if you are, and these symptoms then disappear, you may want to seek advice from your caregiver, as this may be a sign of a pregnancy complication.

Make sure you pay attention to anything that could put your baby at risk, such as drinking too much alcohol (see page 14).

Baby

Shaped almost like a dumbbell, the embryo, at a gestational age of three weeks, has a groove down her back which seals up to form the neural tube. On both sides of this tube, specialised tissues known as somites arise, which will become muscle and other structures. A bulge is beginning to develop where your baby's heart will be and rudimentary blood vessels are growing into place. At this stage the yolk sac (rather than the placenta) provides nutrients and produces blood and sex cells.

Support structures

As the primitive embryo floats within her amniotic sac, her umbilical cord is attaching to the placenta (lower left) so that nutrients must be supplied by her yolk sac (centre).

Make an appointment this week to visit your doctor and confirm your pregnancy, if you like. If you are pregnant, you can schedule your first antenatal visit.

DATES FOR YOUR DIARY

MONDAY	TUESDAY	WEDNESDAY	THURSDAY	FRIDAY	SATURDAY/SUNDAY

FINDING OUT YOU'RE PREGNANT

Sometimes women know instinctively when they are pregnant. This may be due to the almost immediate surge in oestrogen, prolonged high levels of progesterone, and the presence of the pregnancy hormone, human chorionic gonadotropin (hCG), which starts production about a week after conception. Most women, however, take a home pregnancy test. These check the levels of hCG (human chorionic gonadotropin) in your urine. Some tests ask you to hold a stick in your urine flow, others require that urine is passed first into a clean container and then a few drops squeezed from the droper provided onto a window or an oblong stick. Usually, the result appears within minutes and can be read by looking for a coloured line in a window on the stick. You should test the first urine you pass after you wake up in the morning, since this will contain the most hCG.

Early indications

The clearest sign that you may be pregnant is a missed period, although there are other reasons why menstruation may be delayed: stress, illness, extreme fluctations in weight, or your body's adjustment to your coming off the pill, for example.

Tender, enlarged breasts can be a sign of pregnancy; it's not unusual for breast changes to begin a few days after conception.

You may also feel much more tired than usual. This may be due to the high levels of progesterone, a hormone that can have a sedative effect. Fatigue also can result

Performing a urine test
HCG can be detected in your urine four weeks after your last menstrual period. If you think you are pregnant – have missed your period – but the test is negative, you should try again a few days later.

from an increase in your metabolism, which is the body's way of coping with the strain on your vital organs and the support required for the growing embryo. This is why it is important to get plenty of rest.

Wanting to urinate frequently is another common sign as the enlarging uterus puts pressure on your bladder. After about 14 weeks, this will lessen as the uterus rises up into your abdomen.

Changes in taste and smell are normal, too. You may start to feel queasy when smelling or eating particular foods, go off coffee or start to crave a certain food. You may have a strange metallic taste in your mouth.

Your mood might change rapidly, making you overly emotional or weepy; this is due to the action of the pregnancy hormones.

See page 18 for how to deal with fatigue and with nausea or morning sickness, a common early complaint.

EXPECTED DELIVERY DATE

The date of your baby's birth will be calculated 40 weeks from the first day of your last menstrual period (LMP). At 40 weeks of pregnancy, however, your fetus is actually only 38 weeks old (see page 8). Your baby's estimated date of delivery (EDD) is only an approximation, however, and you may go into labour any time between weeks 38 and 42. Less than 5 per cent of babies arrive on their EDD, and women expecting their first baby often have overdue pregnancies.

Mum-to-be

You may visit your doctor this week to confirm your pregnancy (with a blood test) and to get an estimated delivery date. You can calculate this date as 40 weeks from the first day of your last menstrual period (see page 8).

You may notice further changes to your breasts: your nipples may be more prominent and the areolae surrounding them may have darkened, and bluish veins may be apparent just under the skin.

A pregnancy is divided into three periods, known as trimesters. The first trimester is up to week 12, during which time there is rapid fetal development. This is also the time when you are most at risk of a miscarriage (see page 18). The second trimester spans weeks 13 to 27 and the third trimester is from weeks 28 to 40.

Baby

Though just a tube, his heart is starting to beat, and his neural tube is closing in preparation for the development of the spinal cord. His brain is growing to fill his head and pigment is filling the opitcal vesicles, shallow orbs on the sides of his head.

A rudimentary digestive tract begins to form, together with the abdominal and chest cavities. Arm and leg buds have also developed, though an obvious tail is still visible on his curved body. His primitive lungs, liver, pancreas and thyroid gland are starting to develop, his nostrils are becoming distinct and his neck and jaw are developing.

Taking shape

The embryo has a clear top and bottom, and is assuming a characteristic C-shape. His heart bulges and his developing spinal cord is clear.

BABY'S LENGTH AND WEIGHT
His length, from crown to rump, will be around 2–4 mm.
The pregnancy sac is about 2.5 ml in volume.

If you haven't already seen your doctor, ring him or her now to schedule your first antenatal visit.

DATES FOR YOUR DIARY

MONDAY	TUESDAY	WEDNESDAY	THURSDAY	FRIDAY	SATURDAY/SUNDAY

EARLY PREGNANCY COMPLAINTS

Some women sail through the first few weeks of pregnancy without any obvious symptoms. In fact, those who have irregular periods may not even realise they are pregnant for the first few months. Initially, the way you feel may be similar to how you felt just before your period started. For example, you may have suffered from heavy, sore breasts when you were premenstrual. However, nausea and fatigue tend to affect the majority of women to some degree.

Nausea

In the early weeks of pregnancy, the most common symptom is nausea, often accompanied by vomiting. Although commonly called morning sickness, it can strike at any time of the day and occurs more often when you don't eat enough, so always keep some snacks, such as dry crackers or fresh fruit, close at hand.

Dry biscuits
Plain carbohydrates can help to settle your stomach if you feel nauseated.

If you are affected and you usually eat three standard meals a day, try changing your eating pattern to more frequent, smaller meals. Ginger is good for combatting nausea. Use it fresh, adding it to cooking, or take it in tea, as tablets or in biscuit form.

If you suffer from severe nausea, there are various medications that are safe to take and may be helpful, but speak to your doctor before using them.

Because pregnancy heightens your sense of smell, some familiar foods can set off nausea. Common examples are tea and coffee and foods that are high in fat or sugar. Other smells, including your favourite perfume, also may make you feel nauseated.

Tiredness

Most women are surprised at how exhausted they feel early on in pregnancy. Fatigue may be a side effect of the physical changes taking place, including the dramatic rise in hormone levels. You need to get as much rest as you can: go to bed early at night and do gentle exercise to help you relax. Avoid caffeine and sugary foods and concentrate on foods with a low glycaemic index.

PAIN AND BLEEDING

These are not normal symptoms and may indicate a miscarriage or ectopic pregnancy, both of which are medical emergencies.

- It is estimated that 20–40 per cent of all pregnancies end in miscarriage, most in the first three months. Symptoms include heavy, clotted bleeding and cramps.
- An ectopic pregnancy is one where the embryo implants itself outside the uterus, usually in the fallopian tubes. Symptoms include abdominal pain on one side, vaginal bleeding, nausea, shoulder pain and dizziness.

Mum-to-be

Breast discomfort – tingling and heaviness – may be apparent; this is caused by stimulation of the milk-producing glands.

You may also feel irritable, and you'll almost certainly start to feel more tired than previously without extra exertion. This is due to your raised levels of progesterone. Even at this early stage you need to make time for relaxation (see page 34).

You may start having to urinate more frequently and may notice an excess of saliva, an increased vaginal discharge and some unexpected nasal congestion.

Internal changes are also happening – your heart rate rises steeply and your metabolic rate starts to increase – but you may be unaware of these.

Baby

Facial features begin to appear: eyes are pigmented discs on each side of the head; nostrils little openings; the mouth an indentation. Ears are developing on the sides of her neck. Her bumpy head is much bigger than the rest of her body. Arm and leg buds are protruding more and elbows and shoulders are discernible, as are paddle-shaped hands and feet. Her brain has divided into segments and her heart beats at about 150 beats per minute (twice as fast as yours). Muscle fibres are growing in preparation for movement, and her tail is disappearing.

In the lungs, air passageways (bronchi) are forming and the intestines are developing, part of which bulge into the umbilical cord. Her internal sex organs are nearly complete. The umbilical cord is also growing as the placenta matures.

Budding genius

Limb buds and the brain are developing fast. Your baby's head contains some disting-uishing features, such as the eyes. Inside, primitive organs continue to grow, including the liver and lungs.

BABY'S LENGTH
Her length, from crown to rump, will be around 4–5 mm.

Stock up on supplies of ginger, dry crackers and other bland, easy-to-digest carbohydrates to relieve morning sickness.

DATES FOR YOUR DIARY

MONDAY	TUESDAY	WEDNESDAY	THURSDAY	FRIDAY	SATURDAY/SUNDAY

ANTENATAL CARE

You will be seen regularly throughout your pregnancy, though visits to a caregiver and the timing of antenatal tests can vary depending on the GP or hospital and personal circumstances. The chart to the right sets out the range of suitable appointment dates and indicates possible procedures. If you are expecting twins or have a medical problem, you will be seen more often.

Your booking appointment

This first antenatal visit to your doctor or health clinic will usually take longer and be more detailed than subsequent visits. You will be asked about your medical background, lifestyle and family history of things such as multiple births and genetic disorders.

The health of your breasts, heart and lungs will be checked, your abdomen palpated, your cervix examined; your weight and height may be measured. You will have a number of tests (see page 22) and you may be prescribed antenatal vitamins.

Subsequent visits

You and your unborn baby's progress will be monitored. Your caregiver will probably discuss diet and exercise with you, and you should take the opportunity to discuss any problems that may have arisen.

Try not to miss an antenatal appointment – it is vital that your pregnancy is monitored to ensure a healthy baby and safe birth. You may wish for your partner or a close friend or relative to attend visits or tests with you.

APPOINTMENTS FOR YOUR DIARY

FIRST TRIMESTER
Weeks 8 to 12
- Booking appointment scheduled
- Blood testing for genetic conditions may be performed
- Due date estimated

Weeks 11 & 12
- Early/dating scan and nuchal translucency test possible
- Chorionic villus sampling (CVS) possible
- Serum screening possible

SECOND TRIMESTER
Weeks 13 to 15
- Early/dating scan and nuchal translucency test possible
- Chorionic villus sampling (CVS) possible
- Serum screening possible

Week 16
- Antenatal appointment
- Blood test for Down's syndrome may be offered
- Anomaly scan possible
- Amniocentesis possible
- Serum screening including alpha-fetoprotein (AFP) test possible

Week 17
- Serum screening including alpha-fetoprotein (AFP) test possible
- Amniocentesis possible

Week 18
- Serum screening including alpha-fetoprotein (AFP) test possible
- Anomaly scan possible
- Amniocentesis possible

Weeks 20 to 23
- Antenatal appointment
- Serum screening including alpha-fetoprotein (AFP) test possible
- Anomaly scan possible
- Fetal blood sampling possible

Week 24
- Antenatal appointment
- Fetal blood sampling possible

Weeks 26 & 27
- Glucose screen possible
- Fetal blood sampling possible

THIRD TRIMESTER
Weeks 28, 30, 32 & 34
- Antenatal appointment
- Blood test for anaemia and/or glucose screen may be offered
- Fetal blood sampling possible

Week 36
- Antenatal appointment
- Test for Group B Strep may be offered
- Fetal blood sampling possible

Weeks 37 to 40
- Antenatal appointment
- Baby's size and position assessed
- Fetal blood sampling possible

Your antenatal visits
Raise any concerns about your pregnancy at your check-ups; it is a good idea to make a list of things you want to discuss beforehand.

Mum-to-be

Although your uterus is starting to swell it probably won't show just yet. Generally, the only people who will notice at this stage are your doctor – who can feel the enlargement when doing a pelvic exam – and you; your clothes may feel tighter around your waistline. While nausea, tiredness and mood swings are common symptoms at this time and may occasionally prove unpleasant, view them as signs that your body is adapting itself to the demands of pregnancy and the needs of your growing baby.

Baby

His body is unfurling slightly as the spine straightens and his trunk gets longer. His head, bent forward on his chest, is much bigger than his body, and his facial features continue to develop. His arms and legs have become longer and project forwards. At the tips, tiny fingers and toes are growing.

He has a rudimentary nose and tongue and his upper lip is forming. His eyes, with discernible eyelids, are open and spaced far apart, and his inner ears are forming. His heart, brain, liver, lungs and kidneys are now present in a basic form, and his intestines are so long that they are developing outside the abdomen, in a sac adjacent to the umbilical cord.

Head strong

A feature of both a developing fetus and a newborn is that the head is his largest part. Your baby has started to move around, thanks to the firming up and lengthening of leg and arm tissue and the development of his joints.

BABY'S LENGTH AND WEIGHT
His length, from crown to rump, will be around 14–20 mm and his weight is about 3 g.

If your booking visit takes place this week, be prepared for a long visit. Take reading material.

DATES FOR YOUR DIARY

MONDAY	TUESDAY	WEDNESDAY	THURSDAY	FRIDAY	SATURDAY/SUNDAY

ROUTINE TESTS

Throughout your pregnancy your caregiver will perform a number of tests. These include regular checks of your blood pressure and any swelling in your hands and feet and measurements of your fundal height (the distance from the top of your uterus to your pelvic bone). The latter monitors baby's size. Generally, you will only be weighed if you were over- or underweight when you started your pregnancy or if you don't seem to be gaining weight at a reasonable rate.

After week 16 your baby's heartbeat will also be monitored. Depending on your progress, other tests may also be performed (see chart page 20).

Blood tests

A blood test can usually confirm a pregnancy before a urine test. Once you are pregnant, a sample of your blood will be taken to determine your blood group, whether you have healthy haemoglobin levels, are immune to rubella or carry the hepatitis B virus. It also will be tested to see whether you are rhesus (Rh) positive or negative. This last result is very important, because if your baby is rhesus positive and you are rhesus negative, you can form antibodies to your baby's red blood cells, which will have serious consequences for your next rhesus-

positive baby. Luckily, effective treatment is available for mother and baby.

Blood can also be used to check alpha-fetoprotein levels, which can indicate a risk of certain pregnancy complications (see page 36), including fetal abnormalities. You will also be offered an HIV test as part of standard routine tests.

Urine tests

You will have to supply a urine sample at every antenatal visit, which will be tested for protein. The presence of protein in your urine could indicate infection or, more seriously, pre-eclampsia (see page 58). Your urine will also be tested for the presence of glucose, which may indicate gestational diabetes, a type of diabetes unique to pregnancy, in which the body fails to produce enough insulin to cope with the increased blood sugar levels.

Testing blood pressure
Blood pressure is monitored at every visit. An elevated reading may indicate pregnancy-induced hypertension or pre-eclampsia. An average reading during pregnancy is about 120/70.

Mum-to-be

Your body shape will not yet reveal that you are pregnant. The pregnancy hormone hCG (human chorionic gonadotropin) is now at its peak, however, and you will notice certain changes such as your facial skin becoming smoother and plumper, although there may be an outbreak of pimples. You may find that you need to wash your hair less frequently, as it tends to become less oily. Also, your breasts may be fuller or feel slightly tender. At times you may notice some vaginal discharge in varying amounts. This is natural, however, and usually not a cause for concern. If, however, your discharge is very thick and there is itching or a strange odour, let your doctor know, as it may be a mild vaginal infection.

Baby

The embryo looks more baby-like now. Her head is large, her tail has disappeared and her back is straighter; her nose and jaw are complete and her neck is more apparent. A protective membranous lid covers her eyes. Her skin is thickening and hair follicles are developing.

By now her fingers are almost complete and separate, her arms and legs are elongating and she has knee and elbow joints. Her ribcage is closing to protect her heart and her intestines are starting to move their way back into the abdominal cavity, which is now big enough to house them.

Making a move
Although you can't feel anything, your baby is now able to move both her arms (which contain hands and fingers) and her legs (which contain feet and toes).

BABY'S LENGTH AND WEIGHT
Her length, from crown to rump, will be around 22–30 mm and she will weigh about 4 g.

Purchase a properly fitting cotton maternity bra to support tender breasts.

DATES FOR YOUR DIARY

MONDAY	TUESDAY	WEDNESDAY	THURSDAY	FRIDAY	SATURDAY/SUNDAY

BIRTH CHOICES

There is a wide range of childbirth options, including where to deliver and different types of pain relief (see page 74). While it is a woman's right to decide how she wants to deliver her child, sometimes a particular type of delivery may be advised for medical reasons – for example, if you are expecting twins or your baby is in a side-lying or breech position.

Hospital birth

In a hospital birth, there is a 'managed' approach to labour; the mother is cared for by a team of midwives and medical staff. Common practices include electronic fetal monitoring to record uterine activity, inducing the birth, using forceps and caesarean delivery. Usually, there is a wide choice of pain-relief options including epidurals. Some women find managed births reassuring because, in the event of complications, all the latest technology is close at hand. Others, however, find it impersonal and intrusive. Often it is possible to agree upon a more natural delivery procedure with a hospital, so the best of both worlds is available.

Birth centres

These may be independent or part of a larger hospital. Most are run by midwives, with emergency backup available. They are designed for women with normal, low-risk pregnancies and births and offer minimum medical intervention. They aim to re-create a home-like atmosphere and one in which you have more control over the birth, with easy access to a birthing pool, for example.

Home birth

Giving birth in your own home allows you as much time as you need to give birth naturally – without drugs and medical interventions and to have the most control over labour and birth. The birth is usually overseen by a midwife, who can deal with most delivery situations, but is in close contact with a consultant should complications arise.

Throughout your pregnancy, the midwife will see you at home or in a clinic for antenatal check-ups, and to ensure your pregnancy and birth are as risk-free as possible. See page 60 for more information and advice on home births.

Natural birth

Available with many hospital births and all home deliveries, a natural birth is one in which pain relief is achieved through non-chemical means. This could be by controlled breathing; meditation; using labour aids; assuming different positions, such as kneeling, squatting or rocking; or the use of a birthing pool.

The birth of your choice
A homey atmosphere, with dim lights, comfortable chairs and cushions to arrange as you please will help you to relax and gain more control over your delivery. Most hospitals and birth centres have special, sympathetically furnished labour and delivery rooms.

Mum-to-be

High hormone levels will produce emotional as well as physical effects. It is perfectly natural to find yourself getting overwrought or having strange mood swings ranging from feelings of elation to weepiness.

Physical changes include the start of weight gain, potential softening of the gums and a slightly swollen thyroid gland. Because your teeth are now more susceptible to bacteria and plaque, brush your teeth at least twice a day and floss regularly. Arrange to have a dental check, making sure you let the dentist know you are pregnant so X-rays can be avoided.

Now only two weeks from the end of your first trimester, you can look forward to a significant reduction in symptoms such as morning sickness.

Baby

Now known as a fetus (offspring or little one), his body is basically complete. His brain has grown large and his eyes and nose can be seen clearly. Eyelids have fused his eyes shut, which won't open now until week 27.

Twenty tooth buds for his milk teeth are forming in his gums and taste buds on his tongue. Most of his joints, including wrists and ankles, are formed, and separated fingers and toes make him capable of a wide range of movements.

His nervous system is responsive and his fully developed heart beats at 140 beats per minute. His lungs, stomach and intestines are still growing, while the kidneys move into their final position in the upper abdomen.

Hands, nose, fingers, knees and toes

Most of these features are now present in miniature. Soon your baby will start to suck his thumb. Already he can make whole body movements, though only involuntary ones.

BABY'S LENGTH AND WEIGHT
His length, from crown to rump, will be around 31–42 mm and he will weigh about 5 g.

You may get your first 'dating' ultrasound this week (see page 26).

DATES FOR YOUR DIARY

MONDAY	TUESDAY	WEDNESDAY	THURSDAY	FRIDAY	SATURDAY/SUNDAY

EARLY SCREENING TESTS

To check that a pregnancy is healthy and a baby is developing normally, doctors use ultrasound scanning. Should problems be suspected, other, more invasive, tests are available.

Ultrasound

This involves transmitting short pulses of high frequency but low intensity sound waves through the uterus to produce an image of the developing baby and surrounding structures.

The first ultrasound may be performed as early as week 8 of pregnancy, although this varies up to about week 12. The first ultrasound is often called the 'dating' scan because it can reveal the age of the fetus, as well as whether a single baby or twins are present, and the location of the placenta. Later scans will show genitalia and therefore the baby's sex, the position she is lying in, and if there are any developmental abnormalities.

Scans performed in very early pregnancy are usually done transvaginally, using a special ultrasound probe inserted into the vagina. Later ultrasounds are usually performed transabdominally, using a transducer that is moved across the mother's abdomen. In the scanning room, you will be asked to lie on your back next to the machinery and expose your abdomen. The examiner will rub gel on your abdomen that acts as a conductor of sound waves, and will then move a transducer back and forth over the area. An image of your baby will appear on the screen next to you. Most clinics give you a printout of the image for you to keep. The whole process should not take more than 30 minutes.

Nuchal translucency

Ultrasound will be used to check a fluid-filled area behind your baby's neck, which can be used to diagnose the possibility of Down's syndrome (see page 36). This space will be measured and a computer program will provide an individualised risk assessment based on your age and the size of the transparency and in conjunction with certain blood tests. If there is a risk of Down's syndrome or other abnormalities, chorionic villus sampling will be carried out.

Chorionic villus sampling (CVS)

A sample of placental tissue will be obtained by passing a catheter through the cervix or placing a needle through your abdomen. This will be analysed to check for abnormalities of chromosome number or structure or certain specific genetic disorders. It is associated with a small risk of miscarriage. Ultrasound will be used to guide the doctor to the right location and to avoid injury to the baby.

An exciting moment
Ultrasound scanning gives you the opportunity to see your developing baby for the first time. Bone and other dense structures appear white on the screen and softer tissues, such as the heart and kidneys, grey. Ask the technician to point out the different body parts.

Mum-to-be

Your body is now burning up calories at a faster rate than it did pre-pregnancy, as your basal metabolic rate has risen by as much as 25 per cent. The amount of blood being pumped around your body will also increase. This can make you feel much warmer than usual and you will probably perspire more, so drink plenty of fluids.

If you haven't had your first antenatal visit yet, write down any questions you want to ask about your care and your baby's progress. Make sure you check up on your family's medical history, as your caregiver will want to know about anything that could affect your baby.

Baby

All of her vital organs — brain, lungs, liver, kidneys and intestines — are formed and increasing in volume. Her inner ears will finish forming by the end of the week and her eyes, which have moved to the centre of her face, are developing irises. From now until about week 20 she will grow more rapidly. The placenta's blood vessels increase in number to provide her with essential nutrients. Hair and nails are growing and amniotic fluid begins to accumulate, as the kidneys start to function. In her abdomen, the intestines are developing. Part of them still projects into the umbilical cord ('physiological herniation') but they will return to the abdomen next week.

Out of proportion
Your baby's head accounts for half of her body length. This is because her brain gets a head-start during development. The rest of her body will catch up in later months. She can now suck, swallow and yawn.

BABY'S LENGTH AND WEIGHT
Her length, from crown to rump, will be around 44–60 mm and she will weigh about 8 g.

If your doctor recommends a CVS test, it will be performed around this week (see page 26).

DATES FOR YOUR DIARY

MONDAY	TUESDAY	WEDNESDAY	THURSDAY	FRIDAY	SATURDAY/SUNDAY

WEIGHT GAIN

The recommended weight gain for a healthy singleton pregnancy is about 9–13.5 kg and 16–24.5 kg for twins. If you are underweight, however, your doctor may suggest you gain more. If you are overweight, you may not need to gain much weight at all.

Piling on the kilos

At birth your baby will usually weigh under 3.9 kg. The rest of your weight gain during pregnancy, therefore, is made up of the placenta, the amniotic fluid, your increased blood volume and enlarged uterus and breasts.

Pregnant women gain weight at different rates, so don't be alarmed if you get bigger sooner than your pregnant friends. During the first trimester (up to week 12), women tend to gain only 1–2 kg. In the second trimester (weeks 13–27) they gain approximately 6 kg, and during the final trimester (weeks 28–40), about 5 kg. This is just an average, so, of course, your individual pattern of weight gain may differ. At week six there is usually little discernible difference in your weight. You will notice an

increase from about week 12, with the most rapid rise between weeks 20 and 30. After week 36, your weight will tend to remain about level. If you are prone to fluid retention towards the end of your pregnancy, there may be a further increase.

A sudden increase in weight may signify a condition known as pre-eclampsia. Pre-eclampsia can develop into eclampsia and both of these conditions can be life threatening for mother and baby (see page 58). Luckily, however, due to the careful vigilance of antenatal health practitioners, pre-eclampsia is usually detected at an early stage and steps can be taken to reduce the chances of it becoming a serious danger.

Fluid retention

Some pregnant women experience fluid retention during their pregnancy, which will account for part of their weight gain. Fluid retention is most often due to dilation of the veins and pooling of blood, but rarely may be associated with malfunctioning kidneys, heart and liver disorders, or poor circulation.

Exercising frequently and wearing loose clothing can aid circulation. Wearing surgical support hose or stockings may also help.

Watching your weight

Try not to let your weight become an obsession. It is your body's duty to provide a nurturing environment for your growing baby and your increasing weight is a sign of this. In any case, much of the weight you put on during your pregnancy will be lost when your baby is born; breastfeeding (see page 68) can also be helpful for weight loss.

Where the weight goes

Fat deposits for breastfeeding 3.5 kg

Enlarged breast tissue and uterus 1.3 kg

Placenta 0.7 kg
Amniotic fluid 0.7 kg
Baby 3–3.5 kg

Additional blood and fluids 3 kg

Mum-to-be

Your uterus has grown to about 10 cm in width. It is now too big to sit in your pelvis and begins to move up into your abdomen, so if you've had to urinate frequently, this should now ease. Your doctor can predict more accurately your EDD (estimated date of delivery) from your baby's crown-to-rump height, which will be measured on an ultrasound scan.

Although you won't be aware of it, your heart may start to speed up by a few beats per minute, in order to cope with the increased volume of blood circulating in your body.

Any morning sickness should have disappeared – or will do soon. You may have your first antenatal visit this week or some tests; be prepared!

Your baby

Fetal growth continues rapidly – he has doubled in size in the last three weeks, his face looks more human and his organs continue to grow. He is growing hair and nails, and his bones are hardening as calcium is laid down. He is much less at risk of developing congenital abnormalities now.

The pituitary gland, at the base of the brain, is beginning to produce hormones. His vocal chords are starting to form. His digestive system is able to contract to push food through his bowels and he can absorb glucose. Genital organs have begun to form, but only an expert can confirm your baby's sex.

Floating free
Your baby makes the most of his buoyant environment by exercising his arms and legs with a range of fluid and supple movements. He is also capable of a range of facial expressions.

BABY'S LENGTH AND WEIGHT
His length, from crown to rump, will be around 61 mm and he will weigh about 9–13 g.

If you have your antenatal visit this week, ask whether you can stop taking your folic acid supplement.

DATES FOR YOUR DIARY

MONDAY	TUESDAY	WEDNESDAY	THURSDAY	FRIDAY	SATURDAY/SUNDAY

KEEPING FIT

Exercise strengthens muscles, improves circulation, aids digestion and increases stamina, so regular exercise during pregnancy will help combat common pregnancy complaints such as constipation, leg cramps and tiredness. It also helps you to adjust to the inevitable weight gain and prepares your body to cope with the major physical demands of labour. In addition, it releases chemical hormones called endorphins into your bloodstream, which invoke feelings of happiness and relaxation. These endorphins pass across the placenta, so your baby will also feel their positive effects.

Keeping fit throughout pregnancy will increase the likelihood of an easy labour and make regaining your pre-pregnancy fitness levels and shape much easier.

Suggested activities

Gentle swimming and walking are ideal for pregnancy, especially if you were not very active beforehand. Walking increases your circulation and aids digestion, while swimming tones your muscles and increases stamina. Neither of these is likely to put pressure on your joints, made vulnerable during pregnancy (see page 32).

Pelvic tilt

This will strengthen the muscles in the small of your back and help prevent backache. Kneel on all fours with your back straight. Tuck in your pelvis by clenching your buttock muscles and arch your back. Hold for a few seconds, then release.

Antenatal pilates is the perfect pregnancy exercise: it helps improve posture and increases core strength, boosts circulation and helps with fluid retention. Gentle exercises work muscles without straining joints, while the breathing exercises taught in pilates are beneficial in labour and for general relaxation.

Antenatal yoga offers the same physical benefits as pilates, but also aims at improving the health of the mind through various levels of meditation.

Taking care

Be especially careful when weightlifting during pregnancy and avoid any heavy weights; weight training puts pressure on joints and ligaments, which are vulnerable during pregnancy, so consult with your doctor or personal trainer.

Listen to your body and stop your exercise session if you feel dizzy, too hot, too tired or are in any pain.

Most doctors are of the opinion that vigorous sports should not be undertaken in the first trimester, as the risk of miscarriage is greatest then. Although you should seek your doctor's advice first, if you practised a sport such as tennis regularly before you were pregnant, then usually it should not be a problem to continue pursuing it during the first and second trimesters.

Mum-to-be

Now in your second trimester, the best period of your pregnancy may be beginning. You may well find your hunger increases or that you start to crave certain foods or go off others. You will probably start to feel more energetic as first trimester problems, such as nausea and fatigue, ease.

The placenta now produces hormones – mainly progesterone and oestriol – previously produced by your ovaries; these play a vital role in maintaining your pregnancy and inducing the necessary bodily changes.

If you haven't already done so, you can announce your pregnancy now with confidence, as the risk of complications is much less.

Baby

All her vital organs and structures are basically formed, but are still immature. Her intestines have moved further into her body, her liver begins to excrete bile and her pancreas starts to produce insulin. She is also moving constantly, though you can't feel the movements, and bone tissue is appearing. Her reflexes are improving as her nerve cells multiply and neurological development continues apace. If her palm encounters her umbilical cord, her fingers will curl around it.

Your baby has developed opposable thumbs – these are vital tools for all humans as they allow us to pick up, hold and manipulate items.

Front-facing features

Your baby's eyes are at the front of her face and her ears are nearing their final position. She can open and close her lips. Her neck supports her head movements.

BABY'S LENGTH AND WEIGHT
Her length, from crown to rump, will be around 75 mm and she will weigh about 20 g.

You'll probably have had your first trimester scan by now and will want to tell others about your pregnancy.

DATES FOR YOUR DIARY

MONDAY	TUESDAY	WEDNESDAY	THURSDAY	FRIDAY	SATURDAY/SUNDAY

POSTURE MATTERS

Many of the movements that we take for granted – standing, walking and sitting – may need to be adjusted during pregnancy so that you preserve good posture. You need to carry your baby in your uterus in a way that is comfortable for both of you.

Good posture can help to alleviate any unnecessary strain on your back muscles. The hormone relaxin, released during pregnancy, results in softened and stretched ligaments, which can make your back vulnerable to strains. Moreover, as your abdomen enlarges and your baby becomes heavier, you may find yourself leaning backwards or stooping forwards to adjust your centre of gravity. This can strain the muscles around your spine, resulting in backache – particularly during the last trimester.

It's also a good idea to perform some stretches as part of your warm-up and cool-down during exercise sessions; keep your back straight and your body centrally weighted at all times.

Standing

Drop your shoulders so that they are relaxed. Tuck in your buttocks and straighten your back. Lengthen your neck and raise your head as though the centre at the top is being pulled towards the ceiling. Avoid tensing your knees and keep your weight evenly spread between your toes and heels. When at the sink, work at waist height, using a large washing-up bowl on top of the sink if it is low. If ironing, lower the board and sit down to iron.

Sitting

Whether sitting in a chair or on the floor, always keep your back straight. When you sit in a chair, sit flush against the back of the chair so that it supports the small of your back. If your chair doesn't provide this support comfortably, you can place a small cushion or rolled-up towel in the small of your back. To prevent poor circulation, don't sit with your legs crossed and keep them raised whenever possible.

Lying down

Lie down slowly, and always from a sitting position. When you are seated, swing your legs slowly over the bed or couch so that they are parallel with your hips. Gently lower yourself onto your elbows, so they support the weight of your upper body. Using your hands, slide down into a lying position.

Getting up

Raise yourself from a prone (only in the first trimester) or supine position in a series of stages. First, roll onto your side. Next, raise yourself onto your elbows so they support your upper body, and push with your hands to ease yourself into a sitting position. Finally, keeping your back straight, slowly stand up from this position.

Lifting

Squat down next to the item, keeping your back straight. Bring the item close to you then lift it up using your leg and thigh muscles.

Walking

For balanced posture, wear low-heeled shoes and walk with your feet parallel to each other.

Posture check

Look straight ahead and lengthen your neck, keeping your chin parallel to the floor

Relax your shoulders and open your chest

Tighten your abdominal muscles

Keep your pelvis tilted

Ensure that your knees are soft and in line with your ankles

Mum-to-be

At this stage of your pregnancy, your uterus is now swelling week by week. You can follow its progress by locating the top of the uterus – the fundus. The position of this will gradually move up your abdomen over the coming weeks. Lying flat on your back, position a measuring tape at '0 cm' on your pubic bone and count upwards by 1 cm for every week of pregnancy. Your doctor, however, is more likely to monitor the growth of your uterus by ultrasound than by fundal height measurements, as it is more accurate.

If your doctor has advised a CVS or seum screening test (see page 26), it may well take place this week.

Baby

Besides making smoother, more complex movements with his hands, and being able to squint and make various facial expressions, he can now 'suck' his thumb. His nervous system is functioning and he 'practises' breathing movements. It is easier now to determine his gender, as his external genitalia are more developed.

This is also an important week for your baby's developing internal organs and his thyroid gland, which has matured and started to produce hormones. His kidneys are functioning well now, producing and releasing urine into the amniotic fluid around him. His neck is elongating, so that his chin no longer rests on his chest. Head hair is developing and his finger- and toenails continue to grow.

Finer features

Baby's face is now better developed; all his features – eyes, ears, nose and mouth – are recognisable, although his eyelids are still sealed shut. They will open at around 27 weeks.

BABY'S LENGTH AND WEIGHT
His length, from crown to rump, will be around 80–93 mm and he will weigh about 25 g.

Organise antenatal fitness classes and set aside a day for light exercise such as swimming (see page 30).

DATES FOR YOUR DIARY

MONDAY	TUESDAY	WEDNESDAY	THURSDAY	FRIDAY	SATURDAY/SUNDAY

RELAXATION TECHNIQUES

Learning to relax is vital for you and for the well-being of your baby. It is also good preparation for dealing with the physical exertion of labour, when all your muscles will automatically tighten up in response to your uterine contractions and you will need to conserve energy and stay mentally calm.

Some women have difficulty sleeping when pregnant, despite feeling very tired. Even if you don't sleep, just lying down to rest with your eyes closed is beneficial. Daytime naps can help with overall fatigue, and keeping up regular exercise (see page 30) will help you sleep.

Muscular relaxation

Find somewhere quiet, comfortable and warm to sit or lie, then close your eyes. Start by tightening the muscles in your feet for a few seconds, then releasing them. Continue to work from your toes, feet, ankles, calves, thighs, buttocks, stomach, hands and arms up to your face; tighten then release every muscle group in your body. Shut your eyes tightly and scrunch up your brow, then release. Open your jaw wide then release. Now repeat in reverse – work downwards from your face. After this exercise your body should feel pleasantly heavy and limp. Practise at least once a day for 10 or 20 minutes. Combine this with breathing exercises (see below) to intensify the relaxation.

Breathing techniques

It is a good idea to learn some deep breathing techniques while you are pregnant. Controlled breathing will help you to relax and is invaluable during labour, both to deal with the pain and to keep you focussed. Practise regular sessions of deep inhalations through your nose, followed by slow exhalations through your mouth (ten at a time). When you exhale, try to relax your muscles as well. Don't hold your breath, as this makes you tense.

Meditation

Finding a sound or word to repeat, such as the word 'relax', will allow you to block out external sensory input and clear your mind, resulting in mental and physical relaxation and revitilisation. To benefit the most, practise meditation twice a day, for about 15 minutes a time, preferably at the same time.

If you can't find a particular word or phrase that works for you, try focussing on a happy memory or imaginary scene, such as lying on a beach or holding your newborn. Finding a quiet spot, turning off the phone and lying or sitting with your eyes closed make the ideal setting for meditation.

Massage

In addition to the above methods, massage may also help you to relax; ask a willing friend or partner to massage difficult-to-reach areas. Treating yourself to a professional back or full-body massage once in a while can be very rewarding.

Gentle massage
Your partner can help you to relax by massaging aching feet or a painful neck or back.

Mum-to-be

By now your waistband is probably feeling tight, so it's time to think about looser-fitting maternity clothes (see page 38). Constipation may start to be a problem, due to increasing levels of progesterone, which cause the muscles of the intestine to slow, so eat plenty of fibre-rich fruit and vegetables and drink more water.

This week your baby's bones are growing rapidly, so make sure you keep up your calcium intake. See page 10 for information on sourcing vital nutrients from foods.

If you're planning a holiday, the second trimester is the best time to go. Sex may also be back on the menu, as many women find their libido heightened.

Baby

From this week, extra-fine hair, called lanugo, starts to grow over her body, in intricate whorled patterns that follow the grain of her thin, translucent skin – patterns that will later give rise to fingerprints. Lanugo is thought to serve a protective function, acting as an anchor for the waxy skin covering that she will secrete in later months. It will be shed before birth and replaced by thicker, coarser hairs with which she will be born. Hair on her eyebrows and head also continues to grow.

The tiny bones of her middle ear are hardening, but she cannot yet hear properly. With facial muscles developing quickly now, she can make a range of expressions, such as frowning and grimacing.

Skeletal growth

Your baby is producing more bone and marrow, so she is becoming increasingly mobile and flexible. Her arms can now bend at the elbows and wrists and she can make fists.

BABY'S LENGTH AND WEIGHT
Her length, from crown to rump, will be around 9.3–10.3 cm and she will weigh about 50 g.

From about this week onwards, an amniocentesis test may be scheduled (see page 36).

DATES FOR YOUR DIARY

MONDAY	TUESDAY	WEDNESDAY	THURSDAY	FRIDAY	SATURDAY/SUNDAY

FURTHER SCREENING TESTS

Though most doctors prefer to screen for risks of certain genetic diseases as early as possible, certain tests are only reliable later on in pregnancy.

Alpha-fetoprotein (AFP) and triple screen

This blood test is usually performed between weeks 15 and 18 and can determine whether your baby suffers from a neural tube defect such as spina bifida – an opening in the spine which can cause paralysis – anencephaly, a missing brain and skull, or a defect in the abdominal wall. Abnormally high levels of alpha-fetoprotein are indications that your baby may be affected by a problem. This test has a high detection rate, but also has a 5 per cent false positive rate.

A similar test, the triple screen, is beginning to replace the basic AFP test. Also performed between weeks 15 and 18 and known as the maternal screen or MSS, it measures AFP, hCG and oestriol levels.

The quadruple test goes further, measuring the levels of AFP, hCG, oestriol and inhibin, and giving patients an individual risk factor for Down's syndrome. This test is performed around week 16, the results available within a week. Unlike amniocentesis, quadruple test screening carries no risk of fetal trauma. Raise any concerns you may have about any tests with your doctor.

AMNIOCENTESIS

Samples of amniotic fluid can detect chromosomal abnormalities and the baby's sex, which is important if there is a familial propensity for a gender-based disorder. It is usually performed between weeks 15 and 20 and it carries a 0.5 per cent risk of miscarriage. Under ultrasound monitoring, a thin, hollow needle is inserted through the abdomen into the amniotic sac. A small amount of fluid is drawn out to be analysed. The results are available in about 7 to 10 days.

Thin needle

Amniotic fluid

Uterus

DOWN'S SYNDROME

Also known as Trisomy 21, this is a condition where a baby inherits an extra copy of chromosome 21 and, as a result, displays particular mental and physical characteristics. Anyone can give birth to a Down's syndrome baby, but the risk does increase with a mother's age. The probability of giving birth to a baby with Down's syndrome is one in 1,500 at 20 to 24 years old, one in 900 at 30 years old, one in 220 at 35 to 39 years old, and one in 100 at 40 years old.

Fluorescent in-situ hybridisation

This test, also known as FISH, analyses a small amount of amniotic fluid for major chromosomal abnormalities, with the results available within 24 to 48 hours. You can therefore rule out the majority of defects and find out the gender of your baby within 1 to 2 days. However, the amniotic fluid is still cultured, so final results will be ready in about a week.

Mum-to-be

Your uterus is expanding to make room both for your growing baby and placenta and the increasing amount of amniotic fluid – about 200 ml at this stage. Week 16 is an important week for testing: this is when AFP tests and other screenings are usually carried out (see page 36).

In preparation for breastfeeding, your milk glands start production now, which causes swelling and tenderness. Blood flow to the breasts increases, causing veins to become visible and the Montgomery's tubercles (tiny bumps around the nipples) more pronounced.

Baby

Enough calcium has been deposited for baby's bones to show up on an X-ray and his limbs are fully formed, with his legs growing longer than his arms. All his joints 'work' and he can move everything – even bringing up his thumb to his mouth.

His head is more erect and his brain has taken more control of his nervous system and muscles, making each movement more deliberate, rapid and complex. His immune system is starting to produce its own protective antibodies, taking over this role from his mother.

Little acrobat

Now your baby has the space and the ability to practise a wide range of movements. Kicks, somersaults, stretches, twists, turns, wriggles and punches are all attemped, although probably unfelt by you.

BABY'S LENGTH AND WEIGHT
His length, from crown to rump, will be around 10.8–11.6 cm and he weighs about 80 g.

You may be scheduled for an AFP, triple or quadruple test this week.

DATES FOR YOUR DIARY

MONDAY	TUESDAY	WEDNESDAY	THURSDAY	FRIDAY	SATURDAY/SUNDAY

MATERNITY CLOTHES

As your bump starts to grow, you will need to find clothing to accommodate it, and with the huge variety in maternity clothing, there is no excuse to lose your fashion sense while pregnant!

Before rushing out to buy a whole new wardrobe, have a look through the clothes you own already. Any loose-fitting shirts, T-shirts, jumpers and dresses may accommodate an expanding waistline. When your belly becomes more prominent, seek out trousers or skirts with drawstrings or elastic waistbands that sit above or below your bump. Maternity tops and dresses are the most accommodating for a growing belly and can be layered up with a cardigan.

Maternity clothes can often be expensive, so it is worth asking recently pregnant friends and relatives of similar pre-pregnancy sizes if they have any spare maternity clothing.

Shopping for maternity clothes

Most maternity clothes are labelled according to your pre-pregnant size. If you are buying clothes from the non-maternity section, it is best to try on items that are two sizes larger than what you usually wear; you can always add a belt, if necessary.

Always choose clothes that are comfortable and easy to wear. Pregnant women tend to perspire more because of the increase in blood flow, so choose clothes made from natural fibres, such as cotton, wool or linen, which allow your skin to breathe.

Maternity bras

A good quality bra is essential early on in pregnancy. Your breasts start to enlarge very quickly and, if they don't have adequate support, the fibrous tissue will stretch, causing your breasts to sag, and possibly resulting in stretchmarks (see page 46).

Your bra size may well change more than once during your pregnancy, so don't overbuy any one size. It's best to find a bra with at least three adjustment hooks, so that it grows with you. Ensure the straps are wide and the cups soft. Do not wear underwired bras, as these can be damaging to growing breasts. Above all, your bra should be as comfortable as possible, so enlisting the help of a store's professional bra-fitter is wise. If you have very large breasts, you may find it more comfortable to wear a bra 24 hours a day, possibly using a softer sleep bra at night.

Footwear

Wear comfortable, low-heeled shoes that you can slip into rather than ones with laces or buckles. Later in your pregnancy, bending down will get more difficult, so slip-on shoes are best.

Belly bands
Made of thin, lightly elasticated fabric, these bands come in a variety of colours and styles. They sit comfortably on top of your bump and cover flesh exposed when your non-maternity tops start to rise.

Double duty
Many maternity bras are suitable for later breastfeeding, having drop-down cups.

Mum-to-be

To meet the demands of your baby – and the placenta that feeds and cares for her – your heart has increased its output by roughly 40 per cent. This greater volume of blood puts pressure on small blood vessels, such as the capillaries in your nose and gums, so be prepared for minor nosebleeds (and possibly a feeling of congestion) and bleeding gums. You may need to find a bigger bra by this stage and you may find your hands and feet swell a little due to water retention (oedema).

Keep eating healthily, as your baby requires as many nutrients as possible.

Baby

The major step this week is the deposition of brown fat, a special type of fat that will play a big role in heat generation after birth.

Her circulatory and urinary systems are working efficiently now and her heart pumps up to 24 litres of blood a day. Her head is now more in proportion to her body; hair continues to grow on her head and face and eyelashes lengthen.

Matching the incredible growth rate of your baby is that of the placenta. This vital organ develops in tandem with the fetus, from the finger-like projections of the villi in the first weeks, to a 2.5 cm-thick mass of tissue weighing more than 450 g at full term. By week 17 it is large and well established, with a dense network of blood vessels, giving a huge surface area over which to exchange nutrients and waste products.

Delicate complexion
Your baby's skin is still very thin there is no subcutaneous fat to flesh it out as yet. Underneath her eyelids her eyes have grown larger. Her fingers are very well developed and she can do a lot with them.

BABY'S LENGTH AND WEIGHT
Her length, from crown to rump, will be around 11–12 cm and she will weigh about 100 g.

The results of your amniocentesis test may be back by now.

DATES FOR YOUR DIARY

MONDAY	TUESDAY	WEDNESDAY	THURSDAY	FRIDAY	SATURDAY/SUNDAY

SKIN, HAIR, NAILS AND TEETH

Pregnancy hormones often result in a facial 'glow'; skin and nails improve in condition and hair becomes shinier. However, for some women, the high levels of hormones coursing through them may result in more unwelcome body changes.

Skin

Most pregnant women are affected by darkened pigmentation on some area of their body. Body parts already pigmented, such as the areolae around your nipples and any freckles, may become more pronounced. A dark line, the *linea nigra*, may appear down the centre of your abdomen. Although the pigmentation in these areas may stay dark for some time after your baby is born, the colouration will gradually fade.

Dilation of skin capillaries gives rise to spider naevi — raised red marks surrounded by spidery lines. They are caused by elevated oestrogen levels and higher blood pressure, which dilate the tiny blood vessels in your skin and cause them to burst. Red palms (palmar erythema) is a related condition. Again, both of these will fade in time.

Some women find that irregular patches of brown skin appear on their forehead, cheeks, nose and neck. Called chloasma or more commonly the 'mask of pregnancy', it is caused by deeper skin pigmentation. Chloasma is exacerbated by sun exposure, so always use plenty of sunscreen. It usually fades after birth.

Hair

If you're lucky, your hair will increase in thickness, growth and shine. However, some women find that their hair becomes greasy or brittle and falls out in greater amounts. To combat dryness, use conditioner regularly; to prevent breakage, do not brush your hair too vigorously. If hair loss is noticeable, ask your hairdresser about a possible change in style. Hair will improve after pregnancy.

Nails

A common and welcome side effect of pregnancy is that fingernails usually grow stronger, faster and thicker. But if you are unlucky and find your nails get brittle or thin, just keep your hands moisturised and nails cut short.

Teeth

During pregnancy, gums soften and they are more likely to bleed, making you more prone to infection. Make sure your diet contains plenty of calcium and use an antibacterial mouthwash, if necessary. Visit the dentist regularly, but tell him or her you are pregnant so no X-rays are taken.

Mum-to-be

If you're pregnant for the first time, this week can be very exciting as it is around now that you may first feel your baby's movements. Many first-time mothers, however, may not feel any fetal movements until a few weeks later and especially if they are overweight.

Because of the increasing size of your abdomen, you may start to suffer from haemorrhoids (piles) around this week (see page 48). Eating foods high in fibre can help to prevent them and you can ask your doctor or pharmacist about topical creams and ointments to ease discomfort.

Your growing bump may be starting to affect your balance, so take extra care and maintain good posture (see page 32).

Baby

He is more sensitive to the outside world now and signals his presence by means of kicks and prods. His hands can make fists and he should be able to hear, as the part of his brain that receives and processes nerve signals from the ears is developing. He will become accustomed to the sound of blood rushing through the umbilical cord and of your heart beating, but will be startled by any loud noises.

Alveoli (air sacs) are developing in his fast-growing lungs, pads have formed on his fingers and toes and rudimentary fingerprints are apparent. His eyes are in their final position, although still closed, and his face has fleshed out. His lower bowel is gathering undigested debris, called meconium, from swallowed amniotic fluid; this will form his first bowel movement.

If a boy, his prostate is forming.

Little sleepy head
Although he is rarely awake, your baby does have periods of activity when he is able to sense more of the outside world as well as other parts of his body – even grabbing onto his umbilical cord.

BABY'S LENGTH AND WEIGHT
His length, from crown to rump, will be around 12.5–14 cm and he will weigh about 150 g.

If you're seeing your doctor, ask if you can listen to your baby's heartbeat.

DATES FOR YOUR DIARY

MONDAY	TUESDAY	WEDNESDAY	THURSDAY	FRIDAY	SATURDAY/SUNDAY

COMMUNICATING WITH YOUR BABY

You don't have to wait until your baby is born to establish a relationship with her – bonding and communication can begin while she is still in the uterus. At your very first ultrasound scan (see page 26), you may find yourself experiencing strong feelings of closeness to your growing baby, and from about week 18, this maternal-fetal bond grows stronger as your baby becomes familiar with your body rhythms, such as when you eat and sleep, and can be easily affected by your moods. This is why it is important to relax, stay calm and be positive.

Your baby is also very sensitive to external stimuli, so if stroking your abdomen, do so gently. She will also benefit from hearing you and your partner talk to her, or if you sing or play music. Babies who have frequently heard their parents' voices in the womb are more easily soothed by them after birth.

Fetal movements

Feeling your baby move for the first time is an affirmation of your pregnancy, and therefore a very exciting moment. Although fetal movements can rarely be felt before 14 weeks, most first-time mothers feel them between 18 and 22 weeks. However, because

Hearing your baby's heartbeat
From as early as week 14 of pregnancy, your doctor can use a stethoscope or a sonic device to hear your baby's heartbeat.

Fetal bonding
Both you and your partner will enjoy the sensations felt on the surface of your abdomen caused by your baby's movements. Stroking your stomach will reassure baby.

some fetal movements feel like gentle stomach rumblings or butterflies, some first-time mothers might not even be able to identify them until around week 26. Your baby will have her own unique way of moving: some babies are extremely active, others make much more limited movements. As well as obvious kicks and prods, you may be able to feel your baby hiccupping.

As your baby grows, she will take up more of the available space until there is little left in which she can move. If she moves continuously in the same areas, such as under your ribs, this can cause you discomfort.

If the pattern of movements changes suddenly, particularly if they decrease in frequency or intensity, consult your doctor.

Mum-to-be

By now you may be feeling 'the quickening' – your baby's first discernible movements. Other changes include your pattern of weight gain; you may be gaining weight in certain areas, like the buttocks and hips, in addition to the abdomen. Your bigger uterus, together with your extra weight, is probably now affecting your posture, gait and ability to sleep. Try using more pillows for support and to secure a more comfortable position at night.

Baby

Brain growth continues apace. Nerves connecting the muscles to the brain (motor neurons) have grown in place so that baby's movements are now consciously directed. Moreover, these movements are smoother and more coordinated because an insulating fatty nerve coating, known as myelin, has started to grow and promotes the smooth, rapid exchange of information. Your baby's skin has started to thicken, developing four layers.

Special sebaceous glands begin to secrete a waxy substance called vernix caseosa. This is a protective, waterproof barrier for fragile fetal skin that is continuously immersed in amniotic fluid. Any imbibed amniotic fluid is now helped to pass into her circulation for filtering by gastric juices being produced in her gut.

Now, her ears stand out from the sides of her head, permanent tooth buds appear behind the ones for her milk teeth and her limbs are in proportion. Her nipples have appeared and genitalia are recognisable.

Uterine plaything

It is very common to see on an ultrasound scan a fetus grasping her umbilical cord. The thick and knotted texture of this resilient lifeline may provide baby with a variety of sensations to stimulate her sense of touch.

BABY'S LENGTH AND WEIGHT
Her length, from crown to rump, will be around 13–15 cm and she will weigh about 200 g.

You will probably have a detailed ultrasound scan this week or the next to check fetal anatomy.

DATES FOR YOUR DIARY

MONDAY	TUESDAY	WEDNESDAY	THURSDAY	FRIDAY	SATURDAY/SUNDAY

WORKING MOTHER

If you choose to, there is no reason why you should not continue working throughout your pregnancy. It is also a good way to keep busy and take your mind off the long wait! You may find, however, that you need to adjust your work routine for the sake of your own and your baby's well-being.

Safeguarding your health

Different jobs may have certain risks associated with them. For example, research has suggested that very hard physical activity may be associated with a slightly increased risk of compromised fetal growth. Other jobs may pose a risk by exposing a pregnant woman to hazardous substances – a hair stylist, for example, may need to stop working with certain dyes and tints.

If your work involves long hours spent on your feet, you may have to review the situation, as backache is a common pregnancy complaint. Night-shift work may also have to be reviewed, as sleep is increasingly important as pregnancy develops.

Work station set-up

If you sit at a desk all day, you may be at a greater risk of developing a blood clot, so discuss your specific work situation with your doctor. If you work in front if a computer screen all day, take frequent breaks to get up and move around. Make sure your work station is set up properly: sit in a height-adjustable chair with a back rest, wrist support and footstool. When sitting, keep your feet raised as often as possible.

Giving your employer notification

You should supply your employer with a medical certificate confirming your pregnancy – normally by about week 16 – when the chances of miscarriage have reduced. Informing your employer well in advance will give the company plenty of time to make the necessary arrangements for your leave. Your company's policy on maternity leave should be included in your contract of employment – if for some reason it isn't, ask to be given the relevant information.

Pregnant employees are entitled to time off for antenatal care (again, check your company's policies), but, if you can, try to schedule your antenatal appointments around your working day.

All employed women are entitled to (usually paid) maternity leave, as long as they were employed sufficiently long before they became pregnant (currently employed by the same employer continuously for at least 26 weeks into the 15th week before the week the baby is due). Depending on your length of service and your company's policy you may also be entitled to additional maternity leave and pay. Check with your employer, online, the Citizens Advice Bureau or social security office.

Supportive work station
As the weeks go by and your bump grows, you will need to adjust your work station in order to sit comfortably in front of your computer.

Mum-to-be

It is now 18 weeks since conception and you will look noticeably pregnant. Your waistline has expanded considerably so that it is no longer visible and your uterus is pushing your abdomen outwards. At this time, the top of your uterus (fundus) should be just below your navel.

If you have a scan this week, you may well be able to hear the sound of your baby's heartbeat through a stethoscope or Doppler ultrasound – a truly breathtaking experience.

Baby

Now midway into his growth, this time is crucial for baby's sensory development.

More vernix is being produced, anchored in place by the downy lanugo hairs, and is particularly thick around the eyebrows. His skin is thickening and is now four layers, one of which contains epidermal ridges which are responsible for the surface patterns on fingertips, palms of the hands and soles of the feet. Toenails are beginning to grow and scalp hair continues to appear.

If a girl, she now has around six million eggs in her ovaries (though only one million will still be there at birth).

Vital brain development

More of the nerve cells required for the five senses – sight, taste, smell, hearing and touch – have developed. Also increasing are the complex synapses (neurological connections) required for memory and thinking.

BABY'S LENGTH AND WEIGHT
His length, from crown to rump, will be around 14–16 cm and he will weigh about 260 g.

You may be having your second trimester scan or an AFP test this week (see page 36).

DATES FOR YOUR DIARY

MONDAY	TUESDAY	WEDNESDAY	THURSDAY	FRIDAY	SATURDAY/SUNDAY

COMMON COMPLAINTS

The hormonal and physical changes your body undergoes during pregnancy can lead to a variety of physical complaints, the majority of which may be uncomfortable, but are generally not serious. The chart on the right has solutions to some of the most common problems.

Your changing hormone levels can also result in mood swings, including feelings of irritability and anxiety. Controlled breathing and meditation are two effective ways of relaxing and calming the mind (see page 34). Mood swings may be a result of, or accompanied by, insomnia.

Stretch marks

Though not an inevitable result of pregnancy, many women find they develop stretch marks on their stomachs, hips and breasts. These red or brown streaks are the result of a sudden gain in weight. When you gain a lot of weight in a short space of time, your skin doesn't have the chance to adapt and it stretches to accommodate your new shape. While these marks will gradually fade to a silvery sheen, there are things you can do to help prevent them appearing in the first place. The first is to avoid gaining too much weight; if you eat sensibly, this shouldn't be a problem. Keep your skin supple by massaging cocoa butter or almond oil extract into your breasts, hips and stomach. Make sure your breasts are adequately supported; wear a well-fitting bra and, if they are large, wear a sleep bra at night.

Swollen hands, feet and ankles

Normal body fluids increase in pregnancy and about 75 per cent of pregnant women will develop oedema (swelling) at some time. It is most notable at the end of the day, in warmer weather or after prolonged standing and sitting. To help prevent water retention, wear loose-fitting clothing and slip-on shoes and remove any tight bracelets or rings. Don't stand or sit for too long in one position. Sudden swelling may signal pre-eclampsia (see page 58); if this happens, contact your doctor at once.

PROBLEM	WHAT TO DO
Backache	Ask your partner or a friend to massage your lower back. Wear low-heeled shoes throughout your pregnancy and always pay attention to your posture, especially when lifting objects from the floor (see page 32).
Constipation	Drink at least eight (225 ml) glasses of fluid a day. Eat plenty of high-fibre foods, such as fresh vegetables and wholegrain cereals. Frequent exercise (see page 30) will stimulate the digestive tract.
Dizziness	Sit on a chair and bend over so your head is between your knees. When lying down, keep your feet raised higher than your head.
Heartburn	Avoid overfilling your stomach by eating little and often, instead of three large meals. Talk to your doctor about safe antacid medications.
Leg Cramps	To help ease the pain, walk about in bare feet and try stretching and extending your legs and feet. Giving your legs a massage can also help.
Wind and Bloating	Avoid eating large meals that may leave you feeling bloated and uncomfortable. Don't rush your meals; this can cause you to swallow air, which can cause painful pockets of wind.
Varicose Veins	Rest and elevate your legs and feet as much as possible and massage gently around the area – not directly on the veins. Wear support tights.
Breathlessness	Try not to panic if you can't catch your breath as this can make matters worse. Stand tall and allow your chest plenty of room to expand. Try to relax as much as possible and avoid situations you know to be stressful. If you begin to wheeze, experience chest pain or if your fingers and lips turn blue, see your doctor right away.

Mum-to-be

Your weight begins to increase more rapidly over the next ten weeks as your baby lays down her fat layers. This weight gain will be about half your total gain. You may also notice an increase in appetite, prompted by the extra calories you need to support your increased basal metabolism. Continue to eat well but avoid bingeing on one or two foods alone, especially unhealthy and fatty snacks with little nutritional value.

Don't be surprised if you experience a craving for something uncommon. This is known as pica, and soot and soil are among some of the more unusual things for which women have been known to feel a strong desire!

Varicose veins (see page 46) are a potential problem now, so minimise the risk by wearing supportive tights, exercising daily and elevating your legs as much as possible.

Baby

Weight gain continues this week, which is vital for keeping her warm after birth. Her digestive system is now advanced enough to absorb water and sugars from the amniotic fluid that she swallows, filtering some of it through the kidneys and passing what little solid matter there is as far as the large bowel. What her kidneys can't remove is redirected via the placenta to your bloodstream and kidneys. Taste buds are starting to form on her tongue and her sense of touch is improved due to brain and nerve-ending development. On a scan she may be seen stroking her face, sucking her thumb or playing with her umbilical cord.

Sound equipment

Hearing is a feature from early in pregnancy; the uterus is not a quiet place. Your baby hears your voice – including sneezes and coughs, your heartbeat, your organs and circulation 'working', and any hiccups you may make. Soon, your baby will listen all the time.

BABY'S LENGTH AND WEIGHT
Her length, from crown to rump, will be around 18 cm and she will weigh about 300 g.

This could be a good time to buy a baby name book.

DATES FOR YOUR DIARY

MONDAY	TUESDAY	WEDNESDAY	THURSDAY	FRIDAY	SATURDAY/SUNDAY

MORE COMMON COMPLAINTS

Difficulty sleeping

Anxieties about baby's well-being as well as physical discomforts can result in sleepless nights. To help ensure a good night's sleep, have a soothing aromatic bath using a little lavender oil before going to bed. Make sure your bedroom is neither too warm nor too cool and always wear lightweight, unrestrictive nightwear, preferably in natural fibres. Spend time outdoors so you get plenty of fresh air. Don't eat a heavy meal before bed but try a warm drink of camomile tea or milk for their soporific effects.

Haemorrhoids

Many pregnant women suffer from haemorrhoids (piles), usually from around week 18 of pregnancy. Haemorrhoids are swollen (varicose) veins, which appear inside the rectum and may protrude through the anus. They are caused by your growing uterus bearing down on your rectum. The increased pressure impedes the flow of blood in the veins. The veins then dilate to accommodate the trapped blood. The area around your anus may become sore and itchy and you may also notice bleeding when passing stools. To relieve itching, apply an ice pack or some soothing ointment or cream recommended by your doctor. Haemorrhoids usually disappear after delivery.

Frequency of urination

Your growing baby will put pressure on your bladder, which can make you need to urinate more frequently or even leak urine – particularly when you laugh or sneeze. Pelvic floor exercises will help to prevent leakage and

Leg and calf cramps

A firm massage will relieve painful cramps in your calf or thigh. When standing, pull up your foot from the toes and push down into the heel. Briskly rub the calf. If you tend to suffer from frequent cramps, you may be lacking in calcium or salt.

PELVIC FLOOR (KEGEL) EXERCISES

A group of muscles support the openings to the urethra, vagina and rectum. Special exercises will help tone these muscles, enabling them to support your growing baby's weight and helping to push him out during delivery. Keeping these muscles in shape will also help you recover more quickly after the birth. Kegel (so-named for the doctor who developed them) exercises can be done anywhere, anytime and without any special equipment.

To perform Kegel exercises, simply tighten your pelvic floor muscles, hold for a count of five (increasing to 10, 15, etc.) then slowly release. It can help to imagine your muscles as an ascending lift. To make the 'lift' descend, gradually relax the muscles. Repeat as often as possible.

---

wearing light sanitary or incontinence pads will catch any leaks. Although you may be inclined to, don't cut back on your fluid intake as this can cause constipation (see page 46). Urine loss can be a sign of a urinary tract infection and a continuous loss of fluid may be a sign of ruptured membranes; in both cases, contact your caregiver.

Aching legs

Sit in a comfortable chair and elevate your feet as often as possible. Try wearing special support tights or massaging your legs.

Mum-to-be

Your increased blood volume has the effect of diluting your blood to give what is known as the 'physiological anaemia of pregnancy'. Physiological anaemia is common, but your doctor will determine if you are getting enough iron. You can increase your iron intake by eating red meat, bran, sesame seeds and lentils, and accompany with orange juice to aid iron absorption.

Your growing uterus can put pressure on your lungs, stomach and bladder, which can result in breathlessness upon exertion, indigestion and the need to urinate more frequently. Stretch marks may appear on your abdomen, breasts and hips (see page 46).

Now comfortably into your pregnancy, you can think about a weekend break before your bump becomes too big.

Baby

His brain continues to grow very quickly, especially in the area where brain cells are produced, and his internal organs are becoming more specialised in their individual tasks.

Though still red and wrinkled and covered in lanugo, his skin is less transparent and he has developed sweat glands. His fingernails are now fully formed and continue to grow.

Patterns of sleep and wakefulness can now be recorded and your baby is more aware. He can be woken if you tap on your abdomen, by loud noise or by sudden movement. When sucking his thumb, he can either bring his thumb to his mouth or bend his head to his hand. This learning process is repeated after birth, when he will integrate the tactile knowledge he has gained in the uterus with information from his eyes (and from putting things in his mouth).

Gender characteristics

If a boy, your baby's testes are descending from his pelvis to his scrotum and primitive sperm are forming. If a girl, her vagina is beginning to hollow.

BABY'S LENGTH AND WEIGHT
His length, from crown to rump, will be around 19 cm and he will weigh about 350 g.

Think about booking a pregnancy massage or pedicure to give you a lift!

DATES FOR YOUR DIARY

MONDAY	TUESDAY	WEDNESDAY	THURSDAY	FRIDAY	SATURDAY/SUNDAY

MAINTAINING INTIMACY

Sex during pregnancy – penetrative or otherwise – can increase the sense of love, intimacy and sharing between partners. Many women find they have an increased sexual desire during their pregnancy, particularly during the second trimester. This is mainly due to the huge increase in sex hormones (a mixture of oestrogen and progesterone) that start circulating around the body from the moment of conception. As well as heightened sensual feelings, these hormones are also responsible for your hair and skin changes (see page 40). A pregnant woman's blood flow also increases, particularly around the pelvic region, and this makes her genitals more sensitive and easier to arouse. Sex during pregnancy can sometimes be far more exciting than normal and a woman may even achieve orgasm for the first time.

Most men find a partner's changing body extremely attractive. However, there are some men who find the thought of intercourse discomforting because they worry about harming their partner or baby.

Unless otherwise advised by your doctor, there is no physiological reason why you should abstain from sex during pregnancy. Your baby is encased in amniotic fluid, which protects her from any bumps or bruising, and the cervical mucus which plugs the entrance to the uterus prevents any bacterial infections from entering. However, there are things you can do to make the experience more comfortable.

Sex in the 'missionary' position should be avoided after four months; a side-lying or woman-on-top position will allow you to better control the depth of penetration. A lubricant can help prevent soreness and abrasions, and thrusting should be kept to a minimum.

There are also alternatives to full penetrative sex that may be enjoyed by both partners – extended foreplay, sensual massage, mutual masturbation and oral sex, for example. Sharing a bath, kissing and cuddling are other ways of showing affection.

STAY SAFE

Although generally there is no risk to your unborn baby when you make love, you may want to avoid penetrative sex until you are beyond the first 12 weeks if you have a history of miscarriages. You may also want to avoid it in the last trimester if you previously had a premature delivery or are experiencing signs of early labour. You should also avoid sex in late pregnancy if your membranes have broken or if you have any bleeding.

Mum-to-be

Your growing abdomen may be impacting on your digestive system, causing heartburn and indigestion. Eating smaller, more frequent meals can help, as can walking after eating. This may be the time when you start to suffer from anaemia, so it's important to eat plenty of iron-rich foods.

Braxton Hicks contractions may start around now. These irregular and painless contractions are part of your uterus' training for labour. As your pregnancy advances, they will get stronger, but do not mistake them for true labour. You can feel them if you put your hand on your abdomen, but otherwise they may pass unnoticed.

Talk to your baby, as she can hear well now and will respond to various sounds.

Baby

Her face and body look more like a full-term baby now, but her bones and organs are still visible beneath the skin.

Although she is laying down fat at a high rate, she looks wrinkled because skin is being produced faster than the subcutaneous fat that fills it out, so the skin hangs loosely.

Her lips are much more pronounced and her milk teeth buds sit below her gum line. Her eyes – still fused shut – are formed, but the irises lack pigment.

Her pancreas is developing steadily; later it will supply insulin, an important hormone for maintaining fat in her tissues.

Her hearing is more acute as the ear bones have hardened; she can hear deeper male voices more easily than higher-pitched female ones.

Colour change
Your baby's skin now appears red because pigment is starting to be laid down, making the skin colour less translucent.

BABY'S LENGTH AND WEIGHT
Her length, from crown to rump, will be around 20 cm and she will weigh about 455 g.

If you are working, schedule an appointment with the HR department to discuss your maternity benefits.

DATES FOR YOUR DIARY

MONDAY	TUESDAY	WEDNESDAY	THURSDAY	FRIDAY	SATURDAY/SUNDAY

SELECTING BABY EQUIPMENT

Whether you buy new or second-hand equipment, make sure that all items comply with national health and safety standards.

Feeding equipment

For both breast- and bottlefeeding you will need small bottles, rings, teats and caps, a bottle brush and a steriliser. For breastfeeding, you will also need a battery-operated breast pump to express milk, and some breast pads.

Nappies

With fabric nappies, you will need plastic pants, nappy liners and safety pins (unless they are self fastening). You will also need two buckets – one for soiled nappies and one for urine-soaked ones. For disposables, you need nappy sacks and a covered rubbish bin.

Pram, pushchair or sling

Prams are the best, but most expensive, option for newborns.

Sturdy, flat-folding buggies with flat, padded and comfortable seats are also suitable. The seat should face inwards. An umbrella-folding pushchair is only suitable for babies from three months.

A baby sling or soft fabric carrier will enable you to hold baby close to your chest. There are many different styles, but the important thing is that they don't interfere with baby's breathing. The item should carry a safety standards logo.

Car seat

This must be suitable for a newborn and should carry a safety standards logo and ideally have a 5-point safety harness. It must be installed rearward-facing and in a seat not fitted with an airbag.

Bed and bedding

For the first few weeks your baby can sleep in a Moses basket or pram. Later, he will need a separate cot with bars spaced no more than 5.5 cm apart so there is no chance of him putting his head through them. It should have a drop-down side with a safety catch. If purchasing a second-hand cot, check that any woodwork is smooth and there are no splinters, and the paint or varnish is non-toxic. Buy a snug-fitting waterproof mattress.

You will need at least three fitted sheets and lightweight cellular blankets to cover your baby. No pillows are needed: they can lead to suffocation and can cause overheating, a factor which has been implicated as a cause of cot death or SIDS.

Mum-to-be

Your weight gain may be taking its toll and backache, bladder problems, sore feet and general fatigue may all affect you from now on, so start organising things to make your life as easy as possible. For instance, make sure that you continue to wear comfortable shoes and take every opportunity to put your feet up, raising them above the level of your heart if possible. Also, ask your partner, friends and relatives to help with running errands.

You may have an antenatal appointment this week to check on your own and your baby's health.

Baby

This is a landmark week for your baby's growth because, if born now, he might survive. But he is still very thin with immature lungs and would face a catalogue of difficulties. He would need to be kept in an incubator under expert care.

His head is still large in relation to the rest of his body, but his body continues to grow, filling the uterus and making his movements more restricted. He is building up fat but still has red, wrinkled skin, which is thicker on the soles and palms.

Increasingly conscious of the outside world as his hearing is well established, he can hear music, as well as your voice, your heartbeat and stomach rumblings.

Importantly, he has begun producing surfactant, a substance vital in helping his lungs expand at birth by keeping the air sacs from sticking together.

That's my baby!
Your baby's facial features are now more or less complete; his eyelashes and eyebrows are quite well developed and hair continues to grow on his scalp.

BABY'S LENGTH AND WEIGHT
His length, from crown to rump, will be around 21 cm and he will weigh about 540 g.

You should be booking, or at least investigating, childbirth classes now.

DATES FOR YOUR DIARY

MONDAY	TUESDAY	WEDNESDAY	THURSDAY	FRIDAY	SATURDAY/SUNDAY

CHOOSING A LAYETTE

Selecting items for your baby's wardrobe can be great fun, though you should always remember that until your baby is born and her weight and measurements are known, it is best to buy only the immediate essentials – you can always buy more suitable clothing once she arrives. Bear in mind, too, that you may well receive clothes as gifts. In any event, avoid newborn sizes as all babies quickly outgrow these and the same is true when considering more expensive outfits; your baby may only wear them once!

The right choice

Clothes can quickly become dirty or stained, particularly in the nappy area and neckline, so they will need to be changed and washed frequently. Buy colourfast, machine-washable clothes that are also suitable for tumble-drying. Avoid synthetic fabrics, which can be scratchy against your baby's newborn skin; choose natural fabrics such as cotton and wool instead. Organic fibres such as bamboo are also available. Check all garments for raised seams and scratchy labels (you may be able to remove these). Don't buy anything that needs hand washing or ironing.

If you don't know the sex of your baby or you don't want to adhere to the stereotype of dressing girls in pink and boys in blue, then buy items in neutral colours such as yellow, green or white and gender-neutral patterns, such as stripes, plaids, teddy bears and toy blocks.

Until the birth, keep all clothes in their packets with the receipts so you can exchange them if your baby is born prematurely or is very large.

Once baby is here, make sure you wash her clothes before putting them on her the first time. They don't, however, need to be washed separately from your clothes and no special detergent is required either.

WHAT TO BUY

- 50 small-size disposable nappies (to start with) or 24 fabric nappies
- 4 bibs
- 5 vests (with envelope necks and front and back joined by poppers beween the thighs)
- 4 babygros
- 3 nighties (drawstring or popper bottoms)
- 2 hooded baby towels
- 1 face flannel
- 2 cardigans
- 2 shawls
- 1 summer or winter hat
- 2 pairs socks or bootees

Mum-to-be

Your uterus has grown to the size of a football, pushing your diaphragm and lower ribs up, and displacing your stomach. Pressure on your abdomen may cause your belly button to stick out, giving you an 'outie' if previously you had an 'innie'. Together with the effects of progesterone, which slows down the emptying of food from the stomach, the pressure on your stomach means that you are much more likely to back up acid into the oesophagus (lower throat) and get heartburn, particularly after heavy meals.

Baby

She is now well proportioned, though still thin-skinned and skinny. Blood vessels continue to develop in her lungs and her other vital organs are now well developed.

High inside the gums, her permanent teeth are developing in buds and her nostrils are beginning to open. The nerves around her mouth and lips are more sensitive in preparation for breastfeeding and she practises by sucking on body parts.

Sex differentiation is complete: if your baby is a boy, his testes have descended into the scrotum; if a girl, the vagina has finished hollowing out.

Growth time

Your baby has settled into a daily pattern of sleep and activity. It is while sleeping that she develops, grows and prepares for birth. While sleeping, her brain is working, producing rapid eye movements that can be recorded.

BABY'S LENGTH AND WEIGHT
Her length, from crown to rump, will be around 22 cm and she will weigh about 700 g.

See if you can schedule a visit to the hospital or birth centre to check out the facilities.

DATES FOR YOUR DIARY

MONDAY	TUESDAY	WEDNESDAY	THURSDAY	FRIDAY	SATURDAY/SUNDAY

PREPARING YOUR BABY'S ROOM

For the first few weeks, your baby can sleep in a Moses basket or carry cot in your bedroom. This makes his frequent night feeds more convenient for you; it has also been suggested as a preventative measure for cot death or SIDS. However, sooner rather than later your baby should have his own room in which he sleeps and where all his clothes and associated equipment can be kept. Make sure you don't leave all the decorating to the last few weeks when you will tire easily.

Décor

Most people will prepare a baby's room with the intention that he will live there for at least a few years. For this reason, it is important to decorate the nursery in a style that will be suitable when your baby is of toddler and preschool age. Research has indicated that babies prefer bold, primary colours and distinct patterns because they can focus on these much better than soft, pastel patterns. Buy an interestingly shaped or musical mobile to hang over your baby's cot, and large pictures of animals or favourite cartoon characters to put up on the walls.

Furniture

You will need a waist-high changing table with drawers to store nappies, wipes and other cleaning products and other storage units for baby's clothes and toys. Lamps or a dimmer switch on the main light are a good idea for night feeds, as is a comfortable rocking chair in which you can feed your baby. Buy a baby monitor, and make sure that your baby's room is adequately heated (around 20°C), well ventilated and quiet.

Safety

The paint, fabrics and floor coverings you use should be as environmentally friendly as possible. Avoid using any strong-smelling paints, wash curtains before hanging and have someone else remove any old carpet. Careful placement of furniture will make baby care safer and less tiring. Things should be within easy reach for parents, but out of harm's way for baby. Place the cot and changing table against a wall and away from a window; ensure there are no dangling cords from blinds or curtains.

To forestall problems when your baby starts becoming mobile, fit electrical sockets with a child-proof covering and radiators with a protective guard.

Mum-to-be

As you near the end of the second trimester, a number of new discomforts may appear. These include back pain, leg cramps, headaches and pressure on and around your pelvis (see pages 56 and 58 for suggestions on easing these). In addition, your baby's movements may also occasionally cause pain beneath your ribs, which can be relieved if you lie on your side.

Dad may be able to hear your baby's heartbeat if he puts his head on your stomach. A scan at week 26 is a truly bonding experience, as you can see your baby's profile, anatomy, facial expressions and movements.

Baby

Although the space in the uterus is becoming ever more restricted, he continues to grow. His spine is strong enough to support his body and he responds to touch and sound – his pulse quickens when he hears noise and he can move in rhythm to music. He continues to practise breathing movements and his lungs are maturing. His eyebrows are complete and while he still looks lean, fat is being deposited continuously. By the time he is born, his weight will have increased radically and he will emerge rounded and plump.

If a boy, the cells in your baby's testes have increased, which is important for testosterone production.

Touching toes
Your baby can probably hold his feet in his fist now. If he manages to get his feet into his mouth, he will suck on the toes.

BABY'S LENGTH AND WEIGHT
His length, from crown to rump, will be around 23 cm and he will weigh about 850 g.

Discuss with your doctor or midwife your ideas for your birth plan (see page 93).

DATES FOR YOUR DIARY

MONDAY	TUESDAY	WEDNESDAY	THURSDAY	FRIDAY	SATURDAY/SUNDAY

MEDICAL EMERGENCIES

Most pregnancies are without major complications, but things can go wrong so it's important to be aware of the danger signs. Miscarriage, generally as a result of fetal chromosomal abnormalities, is a feature of early pregnancy, as is ectopic pregnancy. The conditions below, while not common, generally affect pregnancy in the second and third trimesters.

Pre-eclampsia and eclampsia

Characterised by raised blood pressure, protein in the urine and increased swelling of the legs and feet, pre-eclampsia affects 6 to 8 per cent of pregnancies, and 85 per cent of these are first-time pregnancies. As well as excessive weight gain, other warning signs are persistent headaches, flashing lights, blurred vision or spots in front of the eyes, or upper abdominal pain on the right side of the body. If you notice any of these symptoms, you should inform your doctor at once. Treatment is directed at lowering the blood pressure. In rare cases, pre-eclampsia can develop into eclampsia and urgent delivery of the baby is generally required.

Incompetent cervix

During pregnancy the entrance to the uterus, the cervix, is kept closed by a plug of mucus. Sometimes, however, the cervix starts to dilate before the pregnancy is complete due to the pressure of a growing uterus and baby. Known as an incompetent cervix, it can result in the amniotic sac sagging into the vaginal canal and breaking, which can bring on a miscarriage. Incompetent cervix is believed to be responsible for 20 to 25 per cent of all second trimester miscarriages.

Securing the cervix
If your cervix opens early, your doctor will put a stitch in it for the duration of your pregnancy.

Uterus
Suture
Cervix

WARNING SIGNS

If you experience any of the following, get in touch with your doctor without delay:
• Unusual persistent abdominal or chest pain
• Excessive vomiting or diarrhoea
• Headaches, flashing lights in front of the eyes, double vision
• Itching all over
• Leaking of blood or fluid from the vagina
• Swollen or painful leg
• Chills and fever
• Painful or burning urination
• Infrequent urination and thirst
• Seizures
• Fall
• Slowing or absence of fetal movements

If it is diagnosed in time, your doctor will put a stitch in your cervix to keep it closed and remove it about a week before you are due. Women at higher risk of cervical incompetence include those carrying more than one baby, or those who have had a cone biopsy, cervical surgery or laser therapy. In these cases, a doctor may recommend a vaginal ultrasound to check all is well.

Placenta praevia

In about one in 200 pregnancies, the placenta lies at the bottom of the uterus instead of at the top. Ninety-five per cent of the time it moves out of the way as the uterus grows, but if it remains in an abnormal position, it can cause complications during delivery. If the placenta blocks the entrance to the uterus completely, a caesarean section will be necessary.

The main symptom of placenta praevia is bright red bleeding, especially after week 28. If this occurs, contact your doctor who will be able to confirm this condition with an ultrasound scan.

Mum-to-be

In late pregnancy the cholesterol levels in your blood rise, but this should not be a cause for concern. Cholesterol is a vital building block for various pregnancy hormones, which are manufactured by the placenta. These include progesterone, which is important for breast development and relaxation of the uterine and other smooth muscles.

Keep talking and singing to your baby, as she knows your voice and will feel comforted by such communication.

Baby

With eye formation complete, her protective eyelashes are also fully grown. She is becoming plumper due to increased fat building under the skin and, if born now, would look almost the same as at full term, albeit a lot thinner and smaller. The taste buds on her tongue and inside her cheeks are fully functioning and she will enjoy sucking on anything that comes within range of her mouth.

Her lungs continue to grow and she would have a 90 per cent chance of surviving if born now. However, she is far from fully developed and would have to be kept in an incubator, artificially respirated. Also, she would have inadequate liver function, an underdeveloped brain and a weak immune system, leaving her susceptible to the sort of infections that a full-term baby would shrug off with ease.

Eye spy...
The long development of baby's eyes is now complete and her eyelids can open some of the time.

BABY'S LENGTH AND WEIGHT
Her length, from crown to rump, will be around 24 cm and she will weigh about 1 kg.

Shop for baby equipment and supplies before you get too big.

DATES FOR YOUR DIARY

MONDAY	TUESDAY	WEDNESDAY	THURSDAY	FRIDAY	SATURDAY/SUNDAY

PREPARING FOR A HOME BIRTH

Risk assessment

Before you commit to a home birth, a community midwife will come and do a risk assessment at your home, checking access and accommodation layout and arrangements for siblings, birth partner(s) and pets. Your and your unborn baby would also be assessed and, if any risk factors come to light, these would have to be resolved before a home birth becomes a viable option.

Which room?

Although you might like to give birth in a specific room, such as the bedroom or living room, it is hard to say where you will feel most comfortable when labour starts. It is a good idea, therefore, to be flexible and prepare a few rooms to ensure that your home birth is a rewarding experience and takes place in a safe and comfortable manner. Your midwife may suggest a downstairs location for the birth if stairways are narrow or twisted.

MIDWIFE'S REQUIREMENTS

- Easy access upstairs, if necessary, as well as to the bathroom and parking, and for emergency services.
- A small, cleared table or large tray on which the midwife can place all her equipment.
- Plenty of towels, face cloths, washbowls and some soft towels or a shawl in which to wrap your newborn baby.

Protection

Because there will be a lot of amniotic fluid and some bloody discharge during the birth, you will need protective coverings for the bed or sofa and the surrounding floor. Alternatively, you can use old sheets, tablecloths and newspapers. You should also stock up on large plastic bin liners to make cleaning up easier.

Comfort

In the bedroom, make sure there is plenty of space either side of your bed for the midwife and your birth partner(s) to attend to you. Gather as many pillows and cushions together as you can and, if you don't already have one, buy a large beanbag. These are all extremely useful in helping you to find a comfortable position during labour. A hard-backed chair to sit on and lean over, or a low stool to squat over, will also be useful. For a relaxed atmosphere, you might also like to have some music and candles.

If you have older children, it is a good idea to have someone come to the house to help look after them, enabling you and your partner to concentrate on your delivery.

Sustenance during labour

You might need some high-energy food to keep you going during labour and, if it is long, you may find that immediately after the birth you are ravenously hungry. Make sure your fridge and cupboards are full before your due date.

Mum-to-be

You are now in the home stretch and will find your relationship with your baby growing as you become familiar with his movements and sleep periods. It is a good idea to 'test' for your baby's movements. During one hour in the morning and evening, you should see whether you can feel at least ten movements. If so, everything is okay. If not, you should contact your caregiver.

Now you will probably start to visit your doctor or midwife every two weeks. You may be offered a glucose screen (for diabetes) and a blood test for anaemia. If you are Rh negative (see page 22), you may receive an injection of Rh immuno-globulin to prevent you from developing antibodies that can cause problems if in future you become pregnant with a Rh-positive baby.

Baby

Now at the start of his third trimester, he weighs about one-third of his estimated birth weight. He continues to make breathing movements, with the fluid entering his main air passageways and not his lungs, and the necessary muscles are developing well. Occasionally he hiccups, which you may feel.

His skin is red and now completely covered by vernix, and his head hair is longer. Subcutaneous fat deposition continues and he is now large enough for his presentation to be determined. This is his orientation in the womb – that is head or breech (bottom) first. Rarely, a baby will be in a sideways or transverse lie.

He hears more and often sucks his thumb or fingers. If your baby is a boy, his testes have nearly completed their descent into the scrotum; if a girl, the labia are still small and don't yet cover her clitoris.

Positioning

If not already in the preferred head-down position for birth, your baby still has enough room to change his position in the next two months.

BABY'S LENGTH AND WEIGHT
His length, from crown to rump, will be around 25 cm and he will weigh about 1.1 kg.

You should be seeing your caregiver every two weeks starting now. Make sure you sign up for childbirth classes.

DATES FOR YOUR DIARY

MONDAY	TUESDAY	WEDNESDAY	THURSDAY	FRIDAY	SATURDAY/SUNDAY

PREMATURITY

Giving birth before your due date can be extremely worrying for parents, as the risk of complications with a preterm baby is naturally higher than for a baby who is fully mature.

What is prematurity?

Any baby born at less than 37 weeks from the mother's LMP is said to be premature. In most of these cases, the baby's organs will not be sufficiently developed and her survival will depend on expert care. Premature babies generally begin life in an incubator in a special care baby unit (SCBU).

What are the risks?

A premature baby is unable to maintain her body heat effectively nor breathe normally. She is at increased risk of neurological, heart, lung and gastrointestinal problems, as well as being more susceptible to infection, as her immune system is not ready to cope with life outside the protective uterus.

Life in an incubator

If your baby is born prematurely (or with a low birth weight), she will be placed in an incubator, which will provide vital warmth; most likely, she will be hooked up to breathing and feeding tubes and a cardiac monitor. Porthole openings in the side walls of the transparent incubator provide access for the nursing staff to care for your baby and enable you to stroke your baby until she is allowed out for you to hold and feed her. If you decide to breastfeed, expressed milk can be fed to her.

Physical contact

Once your baby is ready to leave her incubator, you should be encouraged to provide her with skin-to-skin contact (known as kangaroo care), which has been shown to have many benefits. It makes breastfeeding and bonding with your baby easier, and babies held this way have been shown to gain weight more readily and leave hospital sooner.

Care once home

You will need to have on hand smaller nappies, vests and outfits, as well as a suitable car seat (there are a few models available designed for babies as small as 2 kg). You also may need to adjust your 'nursing skills' when dispensing medications and vitamins, and be able to

Using a sling
A premature baby thrives if freqently in close contact with his mother's body, both naked and clothed.

follow very specific instructions about feeding schedules or caring for ongoing medical conditions.

As premature infants have immature immune mechanisms, you will need to limit holding, touching and close contact to only a few close relatives or friends, and only after they have washed their hands thoroughly; prohibit anyone with a contagious illness from visiting and avoid public places where people are in close proximity. You will visit your doctor frequently to discuss your baby's feeding and nutrition, status of any remaining medical problems and her growth.

There is great variation as to when 'catching up' is achieved. A healthy premature infant usually will have entered the range of normal – in terms of growth and mastery of developmental skills – by a chronological age of 12 to 18 months.

Mum-to-be

You may be leaking colostrum or 'early milk' from your breasts. This is a sticky, watery substance that will provide your baby's first food if you breastfeed. Colostrum precedes the proper milk supply, which may not start for one or two days after delivery. Your breasts are producing this milk under the influence of prolactin, a hormone that is now being produced in large quantities, due to stimulation by your baby.

Your uterus is getting much bigger and now exerts pressure on your internal organs, so having to urinate frequently can be a potential problem when out and about.

Baby

Space in the uterus is cramped but she still stretches and flexes her limbs and sometimes kicks. Her head, which is growing more hair, is more in proportion to the rest of her body as body weight increases. The soft and expandable bones in her skull enable her brain to develop rapidly, and brain tissue continues to grow.

Her brain is now adept at controlling bodily functions such as breathing and body temperature, but if she were born now she would still require an incubator for warmth.

Her senses are more responsive; for example, her eyes have greater sensitvity to the light and she her ability to hear, taste and smell is greater.

Becoming more rounded

Now that your baby has gained weight, she looks plumper and less wrinkled. Her ability to keep herself warm improves with the amount of body fat she lays down.

BABY'S LENGTH AND WEIGHT
Her length, from crown to rump, will be around 26 cm and she will weigh about 1.25 kg.

If leaking breasts are a problem, buy some breast pads or shells to prevent staining to your clothes.

DATES FOR YOUR DIARY

MONDAY	TUESDAY	WEDNESDAY	THURSDAY	FRIDAY	SATURDAY/SUNDAY

PREPARING FOR LABOUR

As your pregnancy advances, it is a good idea to prepare yourself for your labour. Do this by setting aside time to practise certain exercises, which will help you get into suitable birth positions (see page 71) and by making sure you know how to relax (see page 34). Preparations from this week will be especially helpful if your baby comes early.

Squatting

This position is very useful during labour because it enables the pull of gravity to help a baby along the birth canal. Squatting exercises will open your pelvis to its widest and help stretch your perineum (the area between your anus and vagina), which may prevent tearing during childbirth. Unfortunately, squatting is not a position most women adopt during their everyday activities, so it may be difficult at first. Practise squatting by sitting on a low stool: place your feet wide apart and lean forwards, keeping your back straight. Push your knees out wide with your elbows. Once your pelvic joints are flexible and you are comfortable with the position, try to support your body weight without the aid of the stool. You can use door knobs, a sturdy chair or your partner for support. If you can't keep your heels on the ground, place use a rolled-up blanket or towel under them.

Tailor sitting

Sit with your back straight and put the soles of your feet together. Draw your heels up towards your perineum, using your arms to push down on your thighs.

Tailor sitting

This position helps to strengthen the thigh muscles, important for holding squatting positions and improving pelvic flexibility. If you find this position difficult at first, you can use cushions under your thighs as support, or sit with your back straight against a wall. While you are in this position, concentrate on your breathing and relaxation techniques (see page 34).

Daily squats

At first you probably won't be able to hold this squatting position for very long, but if you practise this position for a few minutes every day, then gradually you will be able to increase the length of time held.

Mum-to-be

As you become larger you are probably also becoming slower and clumsier. Remember to maintain good posture when standing and sitting (see page 32). In particular, make sure you always roll onto your side before getting up (from a supine not prone position), because your abdominal muscles have stretched and loosened to accommodate your growing uterus.

As getting up frequently at night to urinate may be contributing to growing fatigue, try to get plenty of rest during the day, and going to bed early – perhaps with warmed milk (which can help you to sleep).

Baby

His lanugo is disappearing so that when he is born only a few patches may be present. His head hair is thicker and his skin less wrinkled due to an increase in baby fat; overall he looks a lot rounder and plumper.

His finger- and toenails are growing fast, his bone marrow has taken over red blood cell production from the liver and his skeleton is hardening more and more. His mimicking of breathing movements is now rhythmic as his lungs are more mature, and he still gets hiccups from swallowing amniotic fluid. Lack of space in the uterus increasingly restricts his movements, but he still kicks – often in reaction to noise. He is awake more often and his eyes open and close more frequently.

If a girl, her clitoris is prominent as the labia are still yet to cover it.

Inner activity

Your baby still has room in the uterus in which he can bring his feet up to his face. Soon, however, he won't be able to do this.

BABY'S LENGTH AND WEIGHT
His length, from crown to rump, will be around 27 cm and he will weigh about 1.36 kg.

Start finalising your birth plan; if necessary, check with the hospital or your midwife about facilities and practices.

DATES FOR YOUR DIARY

MONDAY	TUESDAY	WEDNESDAY	THURSDAY	FRIDAY	SATURDAY/SUNDAY

YOUR BIRTH PARTNER

Giving birth is a powerful emotional and physical experience, and sharing it with someone can make it that much more special. The baby's father is usually a woman's first choice for a birth partner, since he will normally have been involved in the pregnancy from the beginning. However, depending on your circumstances, you may want to ask your mother, sister, close friend or birth specialist (doula) to provide the necessary support.

Before the delivery

Ask your birth partner to attend antenatal classes with you, so that he or she can learn about the changes you are experiencing during pregnancy and the feelings you may have during labour. It is also a good idea to practise labour exercises and breathing and relaxation techniques together, so your birth partner will be able to coach and support you well during labour.

If you are planning to give birth in hospital, you should take your birth partner on a tour of the facilities there so that he or she will be familiar with the surroundings. You should also name your birth partner in your birth 32) and make a note of the role you would like him or her to perform while you are in labour. Your birth partner should also be introduced to your doctor or midwife, preferably before labour begins!

Discuss with your birth partner beforehand the kind of labour you envisage. Since it is impossible to predict just how the delivery will proceed, it is important to be flexible and discuss all the possible options (see page 24). During the birth you may find that you are in too much pain or you don't want to break your concentration to talk. This is when your birth partner should take over communicating your wishes to your caregiver.

Being together

Before the birth, your partner can share in your pregnancy and help with breathing and positional exercises. During the birth, even if you are managing well, the constant presence of a birth partner will be reassuring, helping you to relax and offering encouragement.

Birth partner help during a caesarean

If you have a caesarean birth (see page 82), in most cases your birth partner can be with you in the operating theatre. He or she will stand by your head and should keep you informed of progress. You and your partner should be able to get acquainted with your baby while you are being stitched. However, if you have an emergency caesarean under a general anaesthetic, your birth partner generally will not be allowed in the operating room but will be waiting for you when you wake up.

Mum-to-be

Backache may continue to be a problem as the ligaments and muscles supporting the small of your back relax and loosen in preparation for the rigours of labour. Because your balance is also affected, you should take special care when climbing stairs, walking on uneven surfaces and when out in wet or icy weather conditions.

The average weight gain for a woman at this point in a singleton pregnancy is 8.6 kg. This gain is made up of the baby, the placenta, amniotic fluid, enlarged breasts and uterus, an increase in blood volume and stored fat, protein and water.

You should be thinking about baby's name – and maybe choosing announcements.

Baby

If your baby were born now, her chances of survival have improved this week, because her lungs are better able to inflate properly. This is because there is now more (though not sufficient) protective surfactant.

Weight gain and brain growth continue, and she is almost fully mature except for her lungs and digestive tract. Her eyes are pigmented, though their final colour won't be established until she is six to nine months old. Her eyelids are open during active times and closed during sleep, as they will be in real life.

Almost 450 ml of your blood flows through the uterine wall, and her blood vessels are coming into very close contact with the capillaries of the placenta that carry her blood. Although the two bloods never mix, they are separated only by a very thin wall – the placental barrier – across which water, nutrients and waste are exchanged.

Vital secretions

Your baby's lungs are producing more surfactant. This substance prevents the air sacs from sticking together or collapsing when outside the uterus, enabling her to take in air and breathe properly once born.

BABY'S LENGTH AND WEIGHT
Her length, from crown to rump, will be around 28 cm and she will weigh about 1.6 kg.

At your visits, your blood pressure will be more closely monitored, as a rise in pressure can be a sign of pre-eclampsia.

DATES FOR YOUR DIARY

MONDAY	TUESDAY	WEDNESDAY	THURSDAY	FRIDAY	SATURDAY/SUNDAY

BONDING

You may well be one of those women who immediately falls in love with her baby. But if your emotions don't overflow at first sight, you needn't worry – research has indicated that bonding is not usually an instantaneous process. In fact, most women take time to develop a special, intimate relationship with their baby, especially if the birth was difficult.

Bonding

Most experts believe that in order to facilitate the bonding process, you should spend time cuddling your baby as soon as he is born. Having just emerged from the comfort of your uterus, your baby will most likely be feeling very unsettled, insecure and vulnerable. Skin-to-skin contact will reassure a newborn and will help you get to know your baby.

The more in touch you are with him, the more your feelings will grow, and the happier and healthier your baby will become. This is why it is very important for you to be involved in your baby's care, even while you are in hospital. If your baby has problems and is taken to a special care baby unit (SCBU), you should make an effort to visit him frequently. The sight of your baby in an incubator hooked up to various drips may be distressing for you, but your baby will appreciate the comfort you can provide if you gently stroke him with your fingers, as soon as you are allowed, and softly coo or sing to him.

A father's love

Bonding is not limited to mother and baby: your partner should be involved too. Most hospital staff will give you both time alone sraight after the birth to get to know your baby. If this is not hospital policy, you might like to request this in your birth plan. Fathers often have extended visiting hours, so ensure your partner takes full advantage of these. If your baby is in the SCBU, dad should visit frequently, so your baby maintains contact with both parents. Encourage dad to cradle, bathe and change your baby's nappies as often as possible. Your baby will soon recognise his smell and voice, which is so crucial to the bonding process.

A moment to cherish
Spending time with your baby, breastfeeding or otherwise, will stir powerful maternal feelings and facilitates bonding.

Breastfeeding

This natural process is an ideal way to convey love, as well as sustenance, to your newborn. In addition to nutrients, breast milk supplies antibodies vital for a baby's health, so breastfeeding as soon as possible is desirable. Very few women are incapable of breastfeeding (surgery or disease, however, may affect the necessary underlying structures). A woman's ability to produce milk is not affected by breast size or nipple shape, as a baby sucks from the whole areola and not just the nipple. Moreover, a baby is born with in-built reflexes that ensure she can locate, latch onto and suck from a breast. However, some mothers may need help with technique to be completely successful. If you have problems, seek the advice of a lactation consultant or a breastfeeding organisation such as La Leche League. Your midwife or doctor should be able to point you in the right direction. The sooner you seek help, the more likely you will master the process.

Mum-to-be

This week your growing uterus may trigger a new problem: your baby is probably head-down by now and large enough so that his legs reach up to your ribs. The pressure on them can make your ribcage sore, especially if your baby's feet get caught. Avoid this uncomfortable situation by sitting up straight as often as possible.

Your internal organs can become a little displaced, but this is not normally a cause for concern. Fluid retention, however, may be a problem. It can result in varicose veins and swollen ankles and fingers. Remove any rings from your fingers if they become tight, and don't wear restrictive clothing.

Keep taking antenatal supplements; your baby's demand for vitamins and minerals is especially high just now.

Stay positive – there are only eight weeks to go until you meet your wonderful baby!

Baby

All his senses are complete and in working order, while his limbs and body continue to fill out. His body is now in proportion to his head size. His head hair and toenails continue to grow.

His lungs and digestive tract continue to mature and he practises breathing, which strengthens and develops his lungs. He is passing urine efficiently from his bladder.

By now his head should be down in your uterus, pressing against your pelvic floor, in preparation for birth, which can leave him free to kick at your ribcage.

He sleeps about 90 to 95 per cent of the day (and is probably dreaming), his eyeballs moving behind closed lids.

If a boy, his testes have descended and both testicles are in his scrotum.

Almost ready

Your baby now looks just as he will when born: his face and body have filled out and all his facial features are developed. His eyes are open more of the time.

BABY'S LENGTH AND WEIGHT
His length, from crown to rump, will be around 29 cm and he will weigh about 1.8 kg.

You may be starting your childbirth classes this week.

DATES FOR YOUR DIARY

MONDAY	TUESDAY	WEDNESDAY	THURSDAY	FRIDAY	SATURDAY/SUNDAY

PACKING FOR HOSPITAL

It is a good idea to prepare all the things you will need for your stay in hospital about a month in advance of your estimated date of delivery. If you go into labour unexpectedly, you will not have time to gather all the things you need and this unpreparedness can cause added stress. Pack all your items in a large overnight bag and store it in a place well known to you and your birth partner. You should also make some contingency plans in the event that you go into labour when away from home. If this is the case, your birth partner (if it is not your partner) needs a spare key to your house to get in and pick up your hospital bag for you.

If you have a caesarean delivery, you will be in hospital for longer; in this case, your partner may be able to bring going-home clothes for you and your baby at a later time.

For your baby

Check with your hospital whether you need to bring supplies for baby, other than a going-home outfit and an infant car seat. Usually the hospital will provide nappies and some formula milk, if you are not breastfeeding.

Useful but non-essential items include a mobile phone (with charger), camera (with spare batteries or charger), reading material, snacks and money for vending machines and parking.

Comfort aids

Your birth partner can use the following to help you relax while you are in labour: pregnancy-safe aromatherapy oils; hot and cold packs or lotions; and wooden rolling (or tennis) balls for back and shoulder massage. Sucking on ice can help relieve pain, so check whether there is an ice-dispensing machine near your room.

IN THE BAG

- Copy of your birth plan
- Dressing gown, nightdress and underwear
- Warm socks
- Breastfeeding supplies: nursing bra and breast pads
- Thick-absorbency sanitary towels
- Toiletries, make-up and hairbrush
- Toothbrush and toothpaste
- Loose clothes and comfortable shoes
- Going-home clothes for baby: vest, babygro, hat and shawl
- Extra bag for taking home gifts and supplies

Mum-to-be

The volume of your uterus has grown 500 times over the course of your pregnancy and amniotic fluid is at its highest level. Physiological anaemia (see page 49) starts to fade as red blood cell production catches up with that of plasma. You may also experience strangely vivid dreams and a more frequent need to urinate. If your baby has assumed a head-down position, you may find it easier to breathe and any indigestion should start to improve.

Baby

Restricted inside your cramped uterus, she still sleeps a lot of the time, dreaming vividly. When she is awake she is quietly alert: listening, feeling, maybe even seeing dim shapes, but, above all, learning, as the billions of neurons in her brain forge literally trillions of connections. She is active, though by now her movements are curtailed to a few strong kicks and jabs.

Her bones are fully developed but soft; she is storing iron, calcium and phosphorous to use in further bone development. The mechanism for controlling body temperature, the hypothalamus, starts to function in her brain, but if born now she would still need to be in an incubator to stay warm enough, and although she makes rhythmic breathing movements, her lungs are still immature and she would struggle to breathe air.

Now fatter with pinker skin, your baby should have settled into her birth position and the doctor or midwife (and you) can probably tell which way she is presenting.

Recognisable behaviour

Your baby will increasingly make more of the gestures of a full-term infant. She can stick out her tongue (perhaps tasting the amniotic fluid), yawn, grimace and, in some cases, appear to smile.

BABY'S LENGTH AND WEIGHT
Her length, from crown to rump, will be around 30 cm and she will weigh about 2 kg.

Make sure you check on your baby's movements each day; ask your caregiver what to look for.

DATES FOR YOUR DIARY

MONDAY	TUESDAY	WEDNESDAY	THURSDAY	FRIDAY	SATURDAY/SUNDAY

LABOUR POSITIONS

When the time comes, your body will probably let you know the best positions for birth. In the past, women were made to stay on their backs with their feet up, which is actually very uncomfortable and fights against the pull of gravity. Some women now choose to be propped up in sitting positions on their hospital beds with their legs wide apart, while others want to move around, squat on the floor or stand upright supported by their partner.

During the first stage

While your cervix is dilating and effacing, you will be experiencing contractions of increasing intensity and frequency. During each contraction, lean against your partner or over a chair or wall. You can also kneel on all fours, in which case it is a good idea to have something cushioning your knees. Between contractions, try standing up, walking or, supported by your birth partner, rocking your pelvis from side to side.

All fours position
This relieves backache by pushing your uterus forwards to take pressure off your spine. Also try rocking your hips from side to side.

During delivery

Give your baby as much room as possible by widening your knees and allowing your uterus to tilt forwards. Like most women, your may not be able to hold a squat position for long periods, so drape an arm around your birth partner and your midwife for support. A variation of this is to kneel down, supported on the bed or floor.

Side lying
This position is good if you have an epidural or when you tire, as it can make contractions more effective and help to slow down the baby's descent if he's coming too quickly.

Mum-to-be

Braxton Hicks contractions (see page 51) have probably become more frequent – they feel like a tightening at the top of the uterus that spreads down and then relaxes. The difference between Braxton Hicks contractions and real labour contractions is that real labour contractions become progressively longer in duration, more painful and do not go away. If your waters break you should call your doctor immediately.

Your weight gain begins to slow, but you may be surprised at how big your tummy has grown.

Baby

The hair on his head continues to thicken. At the same time he is shedding almost all of his lanugo, although the vernix is still thick. His skin is less wrinkled and is getting pinker. His tiny, sharp fingernails reach the tips of his fingers.

His adrenal glands, which are producing ten times more steroid hormone (an androgen-like substance that indirectly stimulates lactation) than a normal adult, are the same size as those of an adolescent. These glands shrink after birth. His bones are hardening, except for those in his skull: these remain flexible to enable him to traverse the birth canal more easily.

His immune system can fight mild infections now – except that his lungs may still need time to develop. He is developing quickly so, if you gave birth now, he would probably have nearly the same long-term outcome as a full-term baby.

As space becomes restricted in the uterus, his movements become fewer but more powerful and sustained.

Preparation for feeding

Although thumbsucking isn't yet connected with satisfying hunger, your baby will practise it because it is a way of exploring things. Once born, he will use his sucking reflex to find food.

BABY'S LENGTH AND WEIGHT
His length, from crown to rump, will be around 32 cm and he will weigh about 2.3 kg.

If you haven't already, you should start your childbirth classes now.

DATES FOR YOUR DIARY

MONDAY	TUESDAY	WEDNESDAY	THURSDAY	FRIDAY	SATURDAY/SUNDAY

PAIN RELIEF DURING LABOUR

All women use one or more pain-relieving strategies during labour. Some women are able to make do with natural forms of pain relief – relaxation and breathing techniques, changes in position, water, acupuncture or hypnosis – but most will use analgaesics and/or anaesthetics. Sometimes fear or anxiety will increase pain sensations, which is why it is important to be aware of the process your body will go through during labour.

Find out your hospital's policy on pain relief and discuss with your doctor or midwife the various available options. You may decide you don't want any pain relief, but be flexible – you won't really know how it feels until you start going into labour.

Gas and air

Entonox (50 per cent nitrous oxide and 50 per cent oxygen) is a fast-acting pain reliever, which you inhale via a mask from a cylinder on a mobile support. It takes the edge off the pain and can be used as and when needed. It does not cross the placenta so cannot harm baby, but it can cause nausea and lightheadedness.

Pethidine

This morphine-derived analgaesic drug relieves pain and helps you to relax. It is injected into your thigh or buttock. The effects can last two to five hours. Some women find Pethidine useful because they can doze between contractions and therefore conserve their energy. It is most helpful when early labour is prolonged and uncomfortable. However, one side effect is that it can cause nausea, so it is often given with an anti-sickness medication, and it can hinder your ability to get up and walk about during labour. If given close to delivery, your baby may be drowsy and slow to feed and interact.

Epidural

This anaesthetic injection works by numbing the lower half of your body. Because you have no feeling, you will need to follow your doctor or midwife's instructions on when to push and pant. After a local anaesthetic is given to freeze the back, a fine tube is inserted between your vertebrae into the spinal cord, and the epidural is administered through it. The tube is taped into place in case you need a refill. An epidural takes about 20 minutes to administer and the effects last throughout your labour as the anaesthetist can continue to give medication any time you need it.

Help with pain

Your birth partner can provide comfort and encouragement but an anaesthetist is required to carry out an epidural and to top it up as needed.

Mum-to-be

You probably feel cramped and heavy, as though you don't have room to breathe, or to take in food. Try to eat small meals at frequent intervals, get plenty of rest and, to avoid swollen ankles and immobility, don't sit or stand in one position for too long. If you are making long car journeys, take regular breaks to get out and walk around.

You should be preparing for your leave of absence from work now if you haven't already done so. Other preparations you need to make include buying some properly fitted nursing bras and attending antenatal classes.

Baby

Fat deposition continues, especially around your baby's shoulders, which are becoming plump and chubby, and there is hardly any room now for her to move around. Babies often have scratch marks on their faces when born from when their arms were held close to their face.

Her central nervous system is maturing and she stays awake and aware for longer periods of time. Her digestive system is nearly complete and her lungs nearly fully mature.

She is still shedding her lanugo, although there may still be some present by the time she is born. Her eyes are blue but this may well change after birth.

Positioned for birth
Baby is low down in the uterus, her head near the cervix and her limbs tightly compressed. When contractions start, her head will push against the surface to thin it out, so opening out the birth canal.

BABY'S LENGTH AND WEIGHT
Her length, from crown to rump, will be around 33 cm and she will weigh about 2.55 kg.

Have your partner make a practice run to the hospital so he/she knows where the problem spots are.

DATES FOR YOUR DIARY

MONDAY	TUESDAY	WEDNESDAY	THURSDAY	FRIDAY	SATURDAY/SUNDAY

INTERVENTIONS

If your labour is induced or it is deemed high risk, or as a routine labour practice in some hospitals, electronic fetal monitoring will be used to continuously check your baby's heartbeat. You may like to discuss the alternatives with your doctor or midwife.

Induction of labour

Labour may be started artificially if your baby is at risk because you are suffering from pre-eclampsia or diabetes, or your placenta is not supplying him with adequate nutrients or you are overdue (see page 86). There are various methods.

Oxytocin

This is a hormone produced naturally by your body, which causes your uterus to contract. You may be given a synthetic form, Syntocinon, in an IV drip. This can cause contractions to come suddenly and more severely than usual, so if you are given oxytocin to induce labour, you may also need additional
pain relief (see page 74).

Keeping check

Many women find the visible signs of their unborn baby's stable heartbeat reassuring. However, the printouts need to be interpreted carefully, so make sure your midwife explains them to you thoroughly.

Prostaglandin suppositories and gels

These are inserted high into the vagina and will soften your cervix so that it starts to thin (efface) and widen (dilate), allowing the first stage of labour to proceed. Prostaglandin suppositories will also stimulate your own natural production of prostaglandin, which causes your uterus to contract. Suppositories and gels are quite safe and your movements are not restricted after the first 30 minutes or so. This means you can walk around while you have one inserted, which can also help to bring on labour.

Artificial rupturing of the membranes (AROM)

Also called an amniotomy, a small plastic tool with a crochet-like hook at the end, is inserted through your vagina into your cervix. The hook ruptures the amniotic sac releasing the water inside. Once your waters break, the pressure within your uterus changes. Your baby's head drops into your pelvis and puts direct pressure onto the cervix, which can help labour to start. If AROM does not induce labour, you may need medication to start contractions; now that your baby is not encased in the amniotic sac, he is at risk of infections entering through your cervix.

Fetal monitoring

In the early stages of labour, you will be fitted with two transducers – one of which has an ultrasound device that picks up baby's heartbeat and the other a pressure-sensoring device, which picks up the strength and duration of each contraction. The transducers are attached by wires to a machine that records the baby's heartbeat and your contractions on a continual printout.

During the later stages, your caregiver may also monitor your baby's heartbeat by placing a Doppler probe up against your abdomen, through which can be heard your baby's heartbeat.

If you are a high-risk case, a small electrode on a wire will be threaded through your vagina and cervix to be attached to your baby's head (or buttocks if he is breech). The wire is connected to a monitor and secured by tape to your inner thigh. The electrode picks up your baby's heartbeat and this again is recorded on a computer printout.

Mum-to-be

The top of your uterus now reaches its highest point, just below your breastbone, so breathing may be uncomfortable and you may get jabbing pains in your ribcage. Your antenatal classes are in full swing and you're probably seeing your doctor weekly. In fact, your whole life is gearing up for the birth. If you feel a bit swamped by it all, remember that it's your pregnancy and you are in charge. You set the agenda for your delivery with a birth plan (see pages 92 and 93), and you decide what sort of pain relief you plan to use (see page 74).

One unfortunate side effect of pregnancy hormones is the synchronisation of your hair follicles. Normally your hairs grow at different rates and so fall out at different times. Now a lot of them will fall out together, probably just after the birth. Don't worry about this, as they will grow back soon!

Baby

He continues to gain weight and has almost reached his birth length, making space in the uterus severely restricted. While he cannot wriggle much, his kicks are forceful. You may be able to see the outline of a certain body part such as an elbow or heel appearing under your skin.

His skull is firm but not hard, with enough give for it to deform slightly when he is squeezing down the birth canal; he may engage this week or next (see page 78).

His kidneys are completely developed and his liver can process some waste. His digestive system and lungs are fully mature; when he breathes, he is able to produce the protective surfactant.

He is awake for longer periods and his range of facial expressions is greater.

Baby face

Your baby has characteristically plump, full baby cheeks, due to a combination of fat deposits and powerful sucking muscles, perhaps honed by several months of thumb sucking.

BABY'S LENGTH AND WEIGHT
His length, from crown to rump, will be around 34 cm and he will weigh about 2.75 kg.

Your birth partner, doctor and midwife should be given a copy of your birth plan by this week.

DATES FOR YOUR DIARY

MONDAY	TUESDAY	WEDNESDAY	THURSDAY	FRIDAY	SATURDAY/SUNDAY

RECOGNISING LABOUR

The exact cause of the onset of labour remains unknown. The most widely held theory is that the baby produces substances that result in a change in pregnancy hormones. But you will know you are in labour when you experience regular contractions. Prior to that, there will be a few other signs that labour is near.

Engagement
Between two and four weeks before labour starts, baby's head will descend lower into your pelvis. Known as engagement, there are some related benefits and minor discomforts to baby's head being lower down. While you'll have more space to breathe, you will also pass water and bowel movements more frequently, have aches in your pubic bones and back, sharp twinges in your pelvis and swollen legs and feet. Pelvic tilts (see page 30) and lying on your left side can help to relieve some of this pelvic pressure.

Nesting instinct
During the last month, you'll find you have a sudden desire to empty drawers, clear out cupboards and scrub the house from top to bottom. This is an inbuilt maternal urge to prepare the home for the imminent arrival of baby. While you want to make the most of this burst of energy, take care not to overdo it.

Mucus plug and bloodstained show
As the cervix softens, shortens and begins to dilate, the mucus plug that has sealed the cervix for most of your pregnancy will be dislodged and a small amount of bright red or brownish mucus known as a 'bloodstained show' usually appears. A show may also appear as a heavier discharge or it may be unnoticeable. If you have a show, contact your caregiver for advice.

Rupture of membranes
The amniotic sac containing the fluid around baby will usually rupture – known as the 'waters breaking' – at some point during labour. Occasionally, however, it may rupture before contractions begin in earnest. If your waters break at home, you need to note the time they break and the consistency (fluid containing meconium would be dangerous), and notify your midwife.

Amniotic fluid is usually clear and odourless, and once the bag of waters has ruptured at term, it will go on leaking until delivery (urine or vaginal secretions may leak from time to time). If you become aware of something pulsing in your vagina after your waters break, this may be a prolapsed cord, so you need to call the hospital right away.

Contractions
At some point, any brief, irregular contractions will be replaced by ones that have a rhythmic pattern and longer length. These contractions progressively contract the upper uterus while stretching the lower part and opening or dilating the cervix. By this mechanism, the powerful upper uterine muscles push your baby through the stretchable lower uterus. Sometimes contractions are felt strongly in the back. If you experience back pain every 5 minutes, call your midwife and go to the hospital.

When to go to hospital
The early part of labour – with cramps, backache, increased urination, bowel movements and vaginal discharge, pelvic pressure and leg and hip cramps – can take hours. If you are able to manage the discomfort, stay at home in familiar surroundings. If the contractions first appear at night, try to continue resting as much as possible. You should leave for hospital when you can no longer ignore the discomfort and contractions are so intense that you are unable to hold a conversation during one, or if the contractions have been regular for over an hour – five minutes apart, each lasting between 45 and 60 seconds. Intense contractions that are less than three minutes apart are often a signal that birth is very near.

Mum-to-be

This week or possibly later if this isn't your first pregnancy, your baby should engage. Her head (assuming she is a cephalic presentation, see page 80) will drop down into your pelvis. You will feel this dropping sensation as an easing of pressure on your ribs and internal organs. Breathing and eating should become easier. Your uterus is now pressing down hard on your bladder, however, so expect even more frequent urges to urinate. If this is your first pregnancy, it is likely to go to full term, but if you have had children before, and particularly if you are expecting twins, you can expect to deliver sooner. The average length of pregnancy for twins is 37 weeks, so be prepared by filling your car with fuel and ensuring that your partner is contactable.

Baby

She could now be born at any time. However, this does not mean that she has stopped growing or developing; fat continues to be laid down at the rate of more than 15 g per day, and myelination (the protective coating) of the neurons in the brain is still in progress (it will continue after birth). She may even grow a little in length this week.

Her immune system continues to develop to protect her once she's born. Antibodies she doesn't produce herself she'll receive from you via the placenta, to give her a temporary boost in immunity for the first few 3months of life (see page 83).

She still spends most of her time asleep, but when she's awake, her eyes and limbs will move constantly, as much as they can in an increasingly restricted space.

Most of her lanugo has disappeared but her head hair is up to 2.5 cm long.

Cramped quarters

Research suggests that a baby triggers labour by producing the necessary hormones in response to being in a restrictive environment.

BABY'S LENGTH AND WEIGHT
Her length, from crown to rump, will be around 35 cm and she will weigh about 2.95 kg.

If you are expecting twins, be prepared. The birth can happen or be scheduled for this week.

DATES FOR YOUR DIARY

MONDAY	TUESDAY	WEDNESDAY	THURSDAY	FRIDAY	SATURDAY/SUNDAY

SPECIAL DELIVERIES

If your baby is in a breech position or you are expecting twins, your delivery will usually need additional medical assistance. More often than not this means giving birth by caesarean but, depending on your situation, it may still be possible to have a vaginal delivery.

Breech delivery

Towards the end of labour, most babies will be lying with their head facing the cervix. The medical term for this is vertex or cephalic presentation. Some babies, however, are in upright positions and will stay that way until the birth. Breech delivery – when a baby is born bottom or feet first – occurs about three times in every hundred deliveries. Sometimes a doctor may try to turn a baby around by gently exerting pressure on the mother's abdomen while she is lying down. This is called external cephalic version (ECV) and is successful about 50 per cent of the time.

Breech babies can be born vaginally, but need to be carefully assisted by medical staff. If there is not enough space in your pelvis, the umbilical cord may become compressed while your baby's head is being born, therefore cutting off his oxygen supply. Also, your baby's

buttocks may not stretch the cervix sufficiently for his head to be born – the head being the largest part of a newborn. This may result in forceps being required to deliver the head. Occasionally, a ventouse (vacuum extractor) will be used. Instead of metal tongs, a soft cup is placed on baby's head and suction helps to pull the baby out.

Breech births, with or without forceps or a ventouse, will necessitate an episiotomy because baby's buttocks won't have stretched your perineum sufficiently. This involves the doctor making a small incision through the perineum to enlarge the vagina. This is done both to accommodate any use of forceps and to prevent tears occurring, which can prove more difficult to heal.

Twin delivery

Sometimes, in a twin pregnancy, the uterus is stretched so widely that labour can start a few weeks before your due date. Quite often, the first baby will be born head first and the second will be a breech delivery. If one or both babies are breech, your doctor may recommend that you have a caesarean delivery. In some cases, the first, usually larger baby, is delivered vaginally and the second, generally smaller baby, by caesarean. There is usually a 5- to 10-minute gap between each birth.

Because there is a greater chance of complications with multiple births, if you are expecting twins, you are quite likely to have continual fetal monitoring throughout your labour and delivery. You also will probably be given an epidural for pain relief, which is will be useful if an emergency caesarean is required.

Assisted delivery

If the mother is having difficulty pushing, or the baby needs to be turned or born quickly, forceps may be used to assist delivery. An episiotomy will be done if forceps are used.

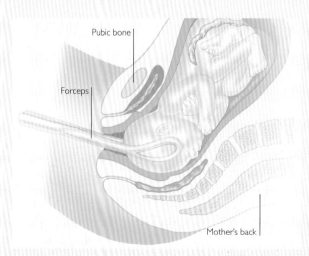

Pubic bone

Forceps

Mother's back

Mum-to-be

Just before your real contractions begin you may experience false labour contractions. Not to be confused with Braxton Hicks contractions (see page 51), these may be nearly as strong as the real thing, but do not become regular and disappear if you move about. How can you tell the difference? If you're not sure, it is unlikely to be the real thing.

Some women may experience a depressed mood, the result of a mixture of anxiety about the birth, fatigue due to a lack of sleep and a desire for the pregnancy to end. If you feel this way, speak to your caregiver and try to focus on the thought that your baby soon will be here.

Baby

Now clinically mature, he is ready to be born. Over the last few weeks your baby has been building up greenish-black waste material, called meconium, in his intestines. It is primarily made up of the products of blood cell breakdown, cells shed by his intestinal lining, and skin cells and lanugo, which have passed into the amniotic fluid and been swallowed. Meconium will be the first waste your baby passes after birth; occasionally it gets excreted before delivery, and the baby arrives covered in unpleasant waste.

The placenta begins to age now, as its role in sustaining your baby comes to an end. It becomes less efficient at transferring nutrients, and blood clots and calcified patches begin to show on ultrasound scans.

Your baby demonstrates a range of facial expressions in reaction to sound, touch and other sensations. Nearly all of his lanugo hair is gone and he is being squeezed by early uterine contractions.

Testicular descent

If your baby is a boy, his testes should now be in his scrotum. By the time he is born, both should be in place.

BABY'S LENGTH AND WEIGHT
His length, from crown to rump, will be around 37–38 cm and he will weigh about 3.1 kg.

If your baby is in a breech position, your caregiver may try turning him with external cephalic version.

DATES FOR YOUR DIARY

MONDAY	TUESDAY	WEDNESDAY	THURSDAY	FRIDAY	SATURDAY/SUNDAY

CAESAREAN DELIVERY

About 25 per cent of all births in the United Kingdom are caesarean deliveries and it is a very safe procedure for both mother and baby.

Reasons for a caesarean

If your pelvis is an unusual shape or disproportionate to the size of your baby's head, your baby will be delivered by caesarean section. Other reasons for a caesarean include a twin pregnancy, placenta praevia, a diabetic mother or a large baby or one in a breech or transverse position. Sometimes, if your labour is not progressing well or your baby has an abnormal heartbeat, an emergency caesarean will be performed to deliver baby quickly.

Procedure

Your abdomen will be covered with antiseptic to kill off any bacteria and some pubic hair may be shaved. You will be given an epidural or spinal anaesthetic (sometimes a general anaesthetic is administered) and an intravenous drip; a catheter will be inserted into your bladder to

The incisions

During a caesarean, two incisions are made – one through the skin and the other through the uterine wall. The cut visible on the outside may not necessarily be in the same position as the internal incision. The cut made in your abdomen usually is just large enough for your baby to be taken out. The most common is the transverse incision: a horizontal cut made across the lower part of the uterus.

Screened off

If you are conscious throughout the procedure, you will be screened from the actual delivery. Your baby will be handed to you after initial birth checks have been made.

empty it. A screen will be placed across your upper body so that you cannot see the operation, but an epidural means you will be conscious to receive your newborn baby, and your partner will probably be allowed to be at your side. The surgeon will make an incision in your abdominal wall and then through your uterus. He or she will then reach in and gently lift out your baby. After an initial examination, your baby will probably be handed to you. He may be slow to respond to his new environment because there has been no adjustment period as there would have been if he had travelled through the vaginal canal.

Meanwhile, the placenta will be removed and examined and your incision will be stitched up. The procedure takes about 30 to 60 minutes, but the delivery itself takes only five to 10 minutes.

Recovery

Because a caesarean delivery is major surgery, it takes a few weeks for full recovery. You will be required to stay in hospital for a couple of days after the surgery – perhaps longer depending on your progress. It may be difficult to sit and stand straight and will hurt when you cough or laugh. Postnatal exercises are necessary to get your abdominal muscles back into shape, but your doctor will advise you on this. To make breastfeeding more comfortable, lie on your side with your baby next to you.

Mum-to-be

Your cervix is ripening in preparation, and your bladder is under more pressure than ever. You're probably nervous about spotting the onset of labour. Strong contractions, that get worse when you move around and become more regular and frequent, are the most reliable signs. Other indications include your waters breaking as the amniotic membrane ruptures and a bloody show as the mucus that plugged your cervical canal is dislodged (in both instances you should contact your doctor or midwife). However, neither of these may happen until well into the first stage of labour.

Baby

Hardly any lanugo will now remain, except perhaps on her shoulders and in the creases of her chubby body. Her toenails reach the end of her toes. The umbilical cord is about 2 cm thick and about as long as she is, and may be knotted or wrapped around her; it is still supplying her with a lot of nutrients as she continues to gain weight.

A few of your antibodies now cross the placental barrier and enter her bloodstream, giving her immune system a temporary boost to help until it gets into full swing. These will disappear within six months.

Head-down position

Baby is almost ready to be born so you could deliver any day now. Space is very limited; baby's limbs are pressed close against her head and trunk and her head is right up against your cervix. This pressure on your cervix will thin the tissues, creating an opening to the birth canal.

BABY'S LENGTH AND WEIGHT
Her length, from crown to rump, will be around 37–38 cm and she will weigh about 3.25 kg.

Time to do an online shop to make sure your fridge and larder are stocked for when you're back home with baby.

DATES FOR YOUR DIARY

MONDAY	TUESDAY	WEDNESDAY	THURSDAY	FRIDAY	SATURDAY/SUNDAY

GIVING BIRTH

There are three stages of birth. The first is when contractions start coming at regular intervals, thinning and stretching your cervix. The second is when you feel the urge to 'bear down' and push your baby through the vaginal canal until she is delivered. The final stage is when the placenta detaches itself from the uterine wall and is expelled.

Transition

This marks the end of the first stage and the beginning of the second. Contractions should now last 60 to 90 seconds and occur at two- to five-minute intervals. Transition is usually the most intense physical and emotional stage of birth. Your caregiver will perform a vaginal examination to see that your cervix is fully dilated (roughly 10 cm) before you start pushing.

Crowning

After transition, you will probably be overwhelmed by the desire to push, and this 'bearing down' is a completely involuntary action. As your baby's head reaches the end of the vaginal canal it will bulge against the perineum, causing some pain and possible bruising. It will also put pressure on your rectum, which can result in involuntary bowel movements. During each contraction your baby's head will start to show through the vagina then recede once the contractions subside. After a few more pushes it will stay there. This is what is known as 'crowning'.

Being born

Once your baby's head has crowned, it will only be a matter of minutes before he is finally delivered. At this stage, you should stop pushing and start panting. This will allow your perineum to stretch and prevent tearing. Now at each contraction, your baby's head will come further out until it appears fully outside the vagina. Once his head is out, your baby will immediately turn it towards the inside of your thigh and the next contraction will probably deliver his shoulders. The rest of his body will immediately slither out, accompanied by a great gush of amniotic fluid.

Mother and newborn
If you request that your baby be handed to you immediately after birth, you may notice that his head is slightly misshapen and that his skin may be unnaturally pale or purplish.

Delivery of the placenta

This can take up to half an hour to be expelled. You may be given Syntocinon, a synthetic oxytocin, which will help your uterus to contract and help reduce blood loss. The placenta is generally delivered with the side attached to the umbilical cord appearing first. It will be checked to see that it is complete and that no placental material remains in your uterus.

Mum-to-be

Try to stay calm while you're waiting for labour to start, and use any false or early labour contractions to practise your relaxation and breathing techniques. Once you go into full labour, it's up to your birth partner to ensure your birth plan is followed (see page 93) but you should be prepared to be flexible, since your labour is unlikely to go exactly according to plan. Be prepared also for labour to be painful. You may have already decided not to use pain relief (see page 74), but you can change your mind at almost any stage.

Baby

The look of a newborn baby is often a surprise for his parents. Firstly, his head may be misshapen, although this rapidly corrects itself within a day or two. Secondly, he may be blue, purplish or pale yellow and he will probably be covered with a variety of substances, including waxy vernix, maternal blood, any remaining lanugo and even bits of meconium if he has passed his first waste in utero. Thirdly, high hormone levels mean that his genitals may be swollen or his breasts might leak a white substance. Lastly, he may have a variety of skin discolourations, spots and dry patches, most of which will eventually fade.

Happy landings
Once the top of your baby's head appears at the entrance to the birth canal, the rest of his head and soon his body will emerge. Changes take place inside his lungs that enable him to breathe.

BABY'S LENGTH AND WEIGHT
His length, from crown to rump, will be around 38 cm (total length 48 cm) and he will weigh about 3.25 kg).

Your baby's size and position will be assessed this week, as he is due to be born.

DATES FOR YOUR DIARY

MONDAY	TUESDAY	WEDNESDAY	THURSDAY	FRIDAY	SATURDAY/SUNDAY

GOING OVERDUE

Pregnancy normally lasts 40 weeks, but you should expect your baby any time within two weeks on either side of your due date. Your pregnancy will only be officially overdue if it lasts longer than 42 weeks. Only five per cent of babies arrive on their due dates, and as long as you and your baby are being carefully monitored to ensure good health, you should be able to continue on with your pregnancy until labour occurs naturally. Many first pregnancies especially go past their due dates.

Risks

If your baby is overdue, she may outgrow her environment and this can cause problems. Her head may not engage properly in your pelvis and your cervix may take longer to efface and dilate, making labour more difficult. Placental function may start to decline, resulting in less amniotic fluid around the baby and a lack of nutrients.

Inducing labour

If your baby is thought to be at risk, you will be induced (see page 86) and some hospitals have a policy of induction after a certain time. But sometimes there are no fetal problems; your baby is just not ready to leave her warm and secure environment, or your due date is inaccurate. Due dates are rarely accurate because they are estimated to be around 40 weeks after the start of the last menstrual period although fertilisation may occur later than mid month. In such a case, you may like to try and bring on labour naturally. Ways to do this include keeping active, gently stimulating your nipples, which encourages oxytocin to stimulate uterine contractions, or making love frequently. However, doctors disagree over the effectiveness of these techniques.

Kick chart

If there is some cause for concern, you can help to monitor your baby's well-being with a kick chart (see right). Printed forms may be provided by your doctor, but you can also make one yourself with graph paper. Mark across the top of the paper the days of the week for three weeks. Choose a convenient 6-hour period (for example, 9 am to 3 pm or 4 pm to 10 pm) to count the number of movements your baby makes, and mark these hours down the side. When you feel your baby's tenth movement during your 6-hour time frame, colour in the corresponding square on your graph. If you notice any change or you cannot count ten movements in the 6-hour period, inform your doctor.

Overdue babies

An overdue baby is called 'post-mature' when her environment has started to deteriorate. Depending on how overdue she is, your baby will look rather different from babies born around their expected delivery date. She will probably weigh more and have no vernix covering her body. This can result in her skin peeling. If she had to use some of her fat stores as nourishment, her skin will be wrinkly and baggy – particularly around her abdomen. She may also have very long fingernails and lots of head hair.

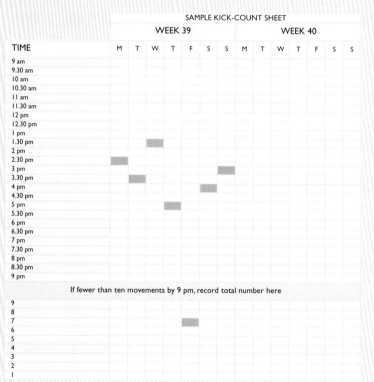

SAMPLE KICK-COUNT SHEET

Mum-to-be

First pregnancies generally extend by approximately eight days; another common reason for lateness is the positioning of baby's head. Depending on your health, being one (or even two) weeks overdue should not be considered a cause for concern. While you wait, your caregiver may perform some tests to make sure your baby is healthy. These include ultrasound scans to check your baby's size and a 'non-stress' test (NST) where your baby's heart-rate is measured. If, however, your pregnancy approaches 42 weeks, your caregiver will probably be discussing induction with you.

Baby

If she is still in the uterus your baby is simply putting on weight, and perhaps getting impatient to be born. If she is newborn, she will find that life is very different from in the womb. Fortunately, she is equipped to cope. Now that her lungs have to provide all her oxygen, a major change happens in her heart. Previously there was a hole through the centre wall of the heart that allowed blood to bypass the lungs, but when she is born, this hole closes up and blood is diverted through the lungs. She also has instinctive reflexes that serve her well, helping her to feed and to bond with you and your partner.

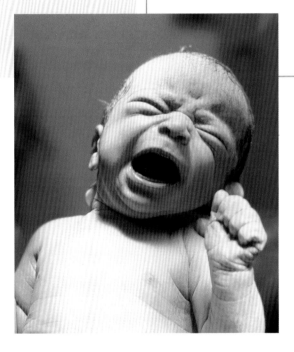

! Think about keeping your phone turned off should baby not arrive and you're tired of telling people this.

Newborn

Your baby will be cleaned up after birth to remove the remaining vernix, blood and other fluids covering her.

DATES FOR YOUR DIARY

MONDAY	TUESDAY	WEDNESDAY	THURSDAY	FRIDAY	SATURDAY/SUNDAY

POSTNATAL BABY CHECKS

As soon as your baby is born, his umbilical cord will be clamped and cut, and he may be placed onto your stomach or at your breast for you to hold and get to know. Although you may prefer him to be handed to you cleaned and wrapped up, immediate skin-to-skin contact helps to facilitate the bonding process (see page 68). He will then be examined to determine his health.

The Apgar test

Named after the American doctor who devised it, this is a series of tests, which all babies undergo immediately after birth and then five minutes later, and can be performed while your baby is right next to you. Your baby's heart rate, breathing, muscle tone, colour and reflex actions will be observed and given a score out of ten. A score of seven or more is normal, so if your baby scores less than seven he may need further examination or special assistance.

Standard checks

These checks will usually occur after you and your partner have had some time alone with your baby. In addition to the ones shown here, your baby will be turned onto his stomach and a finger run along his spine to check for signs of spina bifida. His genitals will be checked for abnormalities. His anus will be examined to make sure it has perforated properly.

Your baby's abdomen will be felt to ascertain the size and shape of his internal organs and to check for any obvious protrusions, which are indicative of an umbilical hernia (a surgically repairable congenital malformation).

Your baby's heart and lungs will be examined to make sure they have developed properly and are performing in a satisfactory manner. Before you and your baby leave hospital, a paediatrician will give him a full examination to confirm that he is feeding well, passing stools frequently and generally progressing healthily.

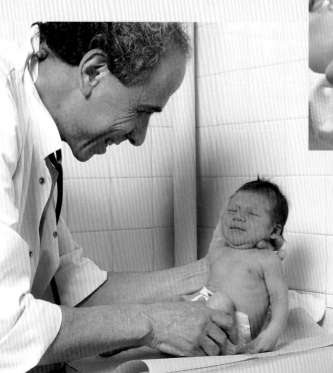

Head and fontanelles

The circumference of his head will be measured and his fontanelles (soft spots on the head) examined. His facial features and inside of his mouth will also be checked for signs of a cleft palate or other defects.

Hips and limbs

Your doctor will bend and circle your baby's legs to make sure there is no hip dislocation. He will also count his fingers and toes.

Mum-to-be

Nearly 10 per cent of pregnancies last this long, particularly for first-time mothers, so don't be anxious if you are still carrying. It may even be that your due date was incorrectly calculated, and you are, in fact, running exactly on schedule. You may prefer to attempt to bring labour on naturally by massaging your nipples – or even indulging in a bout of rigorous cleaning – but health professionals disagree about the effectiveness of such techniques. Talk to your doctor about natural and artificial methods of inducing labour (see page 86).

Baby

Your baby is born with a number of important ingrained behaviours, known as neonatal reflexes, many of which are thought to help him survive. If you tickle his cheek, he will turn towards you to find food; if a nipple, teat or finger is put into his mouth, he will suck on it. If you put your finger in his palm, he will grasp it tightly. In fact, so strong is this grasp that you can lift him from a flat surface. If you hold him upright under his arms and let his feet touch the floor, he will appear to walk.

Reflexes

Babies are born with certain reflexes essential to help them cope with life outside the womb. One of the most notable – yet inexplicable – is the grasping reflex.

If baby hasn't been born, you will almost certainly be induced this week.

DATES FOR YOUR DIARY

MONDAY	TUESDAY	WEDNESDAY	THURSDAY	FRIDAY	SATURDAY/SUNDAY

NAMING YOUR BABY

Choosing a name for your baby can be harder than you think. As well as coming up with something both parents like, the name of your baby will stay with her for the rest of her life, so it must be suitable at all ages.

Choosing a name

As a starting point for discovering which names you like and which you don't, have a look through the numerous baby name books that are available. You should draw up a list of the names you prefer and ask your partner to do the same. Ideally, both of you will have the same name high up on your lists. However, if you have no names in common, perhaps you can find some similar quality. Sometimes a certain consonant (Nicholas, Nina, Natalie), or a theme such as nature (Holly, Ivy, Lily), or old-fashioned names (George, Mary, Florence), will reappear. If you find a commonality, it will give you both something to build on.

When you decide upon a name make sure it sounds harmonious with your baby's surname. As friends will invariably shorten her name, think of all the possible diminutives for your chosen name. If you have a strong dislike of any of them, maybe you could use it as a middle name instead. Check that your baby's initials (middle name included) don't spell an unfortunate word or are the same as her brothers and sisters (this could cause confusion), and remember that any faddish names, unusual spellings, or difficult pronunciation might frustrate your baby for the rest of his life! Names are endowed with sounds, symbols and meanings, and so the name you give your baby may end up playing a great part in defining his personality.

Twin names

Some parents choose names that sound alike such as Hannah and Anna, but other choices could include names that are anagrams of each other such as May and Amy, or those that have the same meaning but are in different languages such as Zoë (Greek) and Eve (Hebrew) for 'life'.

What's in a name...

Choose wisely when you give your baby a name. Bear in mind that she will carry her given name not only during her childhood years, but later on in school and throughout her adulthood. She will be known to future generations by the name you give her, so make sure it is something that will suit all the stages of her life.

Middle names

You might want to name your baby after someone in your family or someone you admire from a distance. Although this can be a sign of respect to the person whose name is being used, it can be a problem if your baby grows up to be nothing like that person. Your child may also feel she has to live up to that person's reputation and you may be disappointed if she doesn't. In these instances it is better to use those names as middle names. There has also been a trend recently to use the mother's maiden name, if appropriate, as a middle name. If your baby has brought together different nationalities then you might also like to reflect this cultural ancestry in her middle name.

Meanings

Almost all names have a meaning and many are derived from the Bible. John, one of the oldest names in English history, is a biblical name that means 'God has favoured' (Jack is a diminutive of it). Others are based on descriptions. Emily has a Germanic derivation and means 'industrious' or 'eager', while Charles means a 'man'. Only a few names, Wendy and Vanessa, for example, are invented and have no inherent meaning.

Name inspiration

Some parents name their baby after a favourite city or country – perhaps their honeymoon location (Brooklyn, Sydney, India, Paris) – or a special time or season, such as when baby was conceived (June, Noël, Summer). Other parents use the arts for inspiration. Shakespearean plays, for example, bring to mind Juliet, Olivia, Orlando and Romeo, while Jane Austen and the Brontës have popularised Emma, Elizabeth, Emily and Charlotte. Other popular sources include Celtic names such as Megan, Gaelic names such as Aiden and transferred surnames such as Clifford.

POPULAR BABY NAMES

Some of the most popular names chosen for babies in the UK in 2010 were:

	BOYS		GIRLS
1	Jack	1	Olivia
2	Harry	2	Ruby
3	Alfie	3	Emily
4	Oliver	4	Grace
5	Thomas	5	Lily
6	Daniel	6	Jessica
7	Joshua	7	Amelia
8	Charlie	8	Chloe
9	Mohammed	9	Isabella
10	George	10	Emma
11	Lewis	11	Lucy
12	Dylan	12	Isabelle
13	William	13	Megan
14	Samuel	14	Ella
15	Ethan	15	Evie
16	Ben	16	Charlotte
17	Jacob	17	Hannah
18	Joseph	18	Ava
19	Luke	19	Holly
20	Ryan	20	Alexa

DEVISING A BIRTH PLAN

Writing down all your thoughts about the way you want to give birth can assist you in identifying some important issues. It is also very helpful to the medical staff if you give birth in a hospital that may have shifts in care. Your birth plan can be written in point form or in paragraphs; what is important is that it briefly outlines your preferences, rather than makes demands. An outline plan is included on page 93. If you prefer not to write your own plan, fill in the blanks on this sample plan. As you may change your mind about what you'd like to happen, photocopy this page before filling it out and then distribute as necessary.

Before you complete your plan, discuss your ideas with your doctor or midwife. Their feedback will give you a clearer idea of what is (and is not) feasible. It's important, too, to discuss your plan with your birth partner – and well before the delivery date. This not only helps to involve him or her in the pregnancy and birth but your partner will then be in the best position to help you achieve the birth you want.

After you write your birth plan you should give your partner and other birth attendants a copy. Make sure you

A COPY FOR YOUR CARER

Discuss your birth plan with your doctor or midwife at least a month before you are due to deliver. As your relationship with your doctor and midwife is an important one, it is better to request your preferences, rather than demand them. Give your caregiver a copy of the plan before hospital admittance.

feel confident that they can convey to the medical staff your preferences in the event that you are unable to.

You should also take a copy of your birth plan with you to the hospital so there is a copy of it with your records. Although most hospitals have certain policies surrounding birth practices, they will make an effort to meet your requests. You need to remember, however, that giving birth doesn't always go as planned, so you should be prepared to adapt your plan and to make some on-the-spot decisions during labour and delivery.

Creating your plan

Writing a birth plan can help you to understand your options in labour and delivery. Your ideas about birth may change as you progress in your pregnancy, so it's a good idea to revise the plan from time to time.

THE BIRTH PLAN OF _____

Where would you like the birth (at home/in hospital or birthing centre)?

_____
_____
_____

How would you like your environment to be (dim lights, music, cushions or birth stool)?

_____
_____
_____

Who will be your birth partner or birth assistant? How do you envisage his/her role – present at all times, actively supportive, informed/asked about decisions needing to be made in the event you are unable to?

_____
_____
_____

What positions would you prefer to be in during your labour and delivery (sitting upright, squatting, active)?

_____
_____
_____

Do you have a preference for a certain kind of pain relief (Pethidine, gas and air, epidural, water), if any?

_____
_____
_____
_____

Do you have any strong feelings about having fetal monitoring (continuous/never, only during certain times, only under certain situations)?

_____
_____
_____

Do you have any strong feelings about the use of forceps or a vacuum extractor (yes/no, only under certain situations)?

_____
_____
_____

How would you like your birth to proceed if you need an emergency caesarean (baby handed to birth partner, type of incision)?

_____
_____

Who should cut the cord, the doctor or midwife or your birth partner?

_____
_____

Do you have any requests if your doctor believes an episiotomy is necessary (would you rather chance a tear)?

_____
_____
_____

Would you like the delivery of the placenta to be speeded up artificially (yes/no) and if so, by what method?

_____
_____
_____

What are your requests regarding feeding (breast/bottle, right away, on demand, daytime only)?

_____
_____
_____

How do you feel about the presence of student midwives/doctors (yes/no)?

_____
_____
_____

How would you like your baby to be handed to you after the birth (immediately, cleaned and wrapped up, after your partner [if you have a general anaesthetic])?

_____
_____

Do you have any strong feelings about the placement of your baby while you are recovering (next to you in a cot, in the nursery)?

_____
_____
_____

Your body will need time to recover from the rigours of labour and/or the trauma of a caesarean. Eating a good diet; engaging in a safe, habitual fitness programme and monitoring your emotions need to be part of the process. Some women prefer to wait until after their postnatal appointment, about six weeks after the birth, before embarking on any programme to get back in shape.

Aches and pains

If you laboured, your muscles may ache and you may have strong pains, similar to period pains, in your abdomen. Known as 'after pains', these are triggered by the release of oxytocin, the hormone that contracts and shrinks the uterus to decrease bleeding after birth. Happily, the discomfort from postnatal contractions decreases each day and can be lessened by taking safe, pain-killing medications such as ibuprofen or paracetamol.

If you had a vaginal birth, your gential area will be swollen, sore and stretched. If labour was long and difficult, or you had a tear, stitches or an episiotomy, you will have pain and discomfort and the perineum (the area between the vagina and anus) may feel quite numb. Try the self-help remedies to help ease the pain.

Lochia

After the birth, blood, mucus and tissue exit through the uterus. Known as 'lochia', this discharge is initially heavy, dark red and thick and may contain large blood clots. It can be particularly heavy when getting out of bed and breastfeeding. Lochia can last up to six weeks, but gradually the flow becomes less heavy and paler. Use special maternity pads, not tampons, to absorb the discharge, and change them frequently. If the bleeding suddenly becomes heavier, turns bright red, contains large clots or smells unpleasant, notify your GP immediately as this could be a sign of infection.

Breast discomfort

The hormonal changes that prime your breasts for breastfeeding take place about two to three days after birth (this is also true if you do not breastfeed). Known as 'engorgement', your breasts will become larger and firmer and may be painful. To feel more comfortable, it's essential you wear a well-fitting, supportive bra, possibly 24 hours a day, until your milk 'comes in' and your

---

SELF HELP FOR PERINEAL PAIN

- Pelvic floor exercises (see page 48) will reduce pain, help you to regain muscle tone after delivery and promote healing by increasing circulation in the area.
- Drinking plenty of fluids dilutes urine so that it doesn't burn as much. You should also empty your bladder regularly.
- An ice pack or bag of frozen peas, wrapped in a soft cloth, can be placed on the perineum for 5 minutes, every couple of hours during the first 24 hours.
- Squat over the toilet, angling your bottom so urine misses the tender spot rather than sitting down.
- Keep a jug of cool water in the bathroom, so you can pour water between your legs as you urinate and when you have finished so that there is no urine left on your skin.
- Sit in a sitz bath (a bowl filled with warm water) or apply warm compresses for about 20 minutes three times a day.
- Soak a maternity pad in witch hazel; it will cool the area and prevent blood sticking to any pubic hair.

---

breasts soften. Before breastfeeding, you may find it helps to put warm compresses on your breasts; the moist heat will dilate the milk ducts making your milk will flow more easily.

If you are not going to breastfeed, try putting a cool compress on your breasts and take an analgaesic such as paracetamol or ibuprofen. Don't stimulate your breasts or try to express milk to relieve pressure, as this will only cause your body to produce more milk. Lack of stimulation by a sucking baby will gradually slow and then stop milk production.

If your breasts become inflamed or extremely uncomfortable, see your doctor.

Getting periods back

Periods generally re-start within four to six weeks, though if you are breastfeeding, periods may be irregular or not appear until you have stopped. The amount of menstrual flow for the first few cycles can range from light to quite heavy, but should soon settle down into a more consistent pattern after that. Ovulation begins again after the first period following childbirth, so having unprotected sex could result in another pregnancy. To prevent this, some form of contraception is needed as soon as you start having sex again. Breastfeeding mothers may be able to take a progesterone-only pill. Those who are not breastfeeding can start taking birth control pills about two to three weeks after the birth. Barrier contraception should not be used if stitches are present or until the cervix is completely healed.

Elimination difficulties

Although it's essential that the bladder is emptied within six to eight hours of delivery to avoid urinary tract infections and to prevent the bladder from becoming distended, which could cause a loss of muscle tone, some women have no urge to go or want to go but can't. You will probably urinate frequently and copiously about 24 hours after the birth to expel pregnancy fluids. To help get your bladder working, drink plenty of fluids and get up and walk about as soon after delivery as allowable.

Although the first few bowel movements may cause discomfort, any stitches won't be affected, and you should be back to normal within a few days. Eating fibre – whole grains and fresh fruit and vegetables – and drinking plenty of fluids will help to get your bowels moving again. Gentle exercise and pelvic floor exercises (see page 48) should help to ease any discomfort. If you become constipated, your GP may suggest stool softeners or a laxative.

Body shape and weight loss

On average, giving birth results in a 5-kg weight loss. Your stomach will stick out due to fluid retention and a distended uterus; your skin will sag because it is overstretched and you will have lost muscle tone. Over time, your body will get closer to its pre-pregnancy shape if you eat a healthy, nutritious diet and make sure you exercise regularly.

Emotional changes

More than half of all new mothers suffer from the baby blues – mood changes; vague sadness; feeling weepy, irritable, anxious and confused – which may occur a day or two after birth and last for about 10 to 14 days. Although the exact cause of baby blues is not known, rapid hormone shifts and sleep deprivation are common suspects, which is why you should nap whenever you can and try some relaxation techniques. Lack of sleep can be a big contributing factor; physical fatigue can reduce the amount of stress you can handle.

INDEX